Mometrix
TEST PREPARATION

Mammography Exam Secrets Study Guide

DEAR FUTURE EXAM SUCCESS STORY

First of all, **THANK YOU** for purchasing Mometrix study materials!

Second, congratulations! You are one of the few determined test-takers who are committed to doing whatever it takes to excel on your exam. **You have come to the right place.** We developed these study materials with one goal in mind: to deliver you the information you need in a format that's concise and easy to use.

In addition to optimizing your guide for the content of the test, we've outlined our recommended steps for breaking down the preparation process into small, attainable goals so you can make sure you stay on track.

We've also analyzed the entire test-taking process, identifying the most common pitfalls and showing how you can overcome them and be ready for any curveball the test throws you.

Standardized testing is one of the biggest obstacles on your road to success, which only increases the importance of doing well in the high-pressure, high-stakes environment of test day. Your results on this test could have a significant impact on your future, and this guide provides the information and practical advice to help you achieve your full potential on test day.

Your success is our success

We would love to hear from you! If you would like to share the story of your exam success or if you have any questions or comments in regard to our products, please contact us at **800-673-8175** or **support@mometrix.com**.

Thanks again for your business and we wish you continued success!

Sincerely,
The Mometrix Test Preparation Team

Need more help? Check out our flashcards at:
http://MometrixFlashcards.com/Mammography

Table of Contents

Introduction

Thank you for purchasing this resource! You have made the choice to prepare yourself for a test that could have a huge impact on your future, and this guide is designed to help you be fully ready for test day. Obviously, it's important to have a solid understanding of the test material, but you also need to be prepared for the unique environment and stressors of the test, so that you can perform to the best of your abilities.

For this purpose, the first section that appears in this guide is the **Secret Keys**. We've devoted countless hours to meticulously researching what works and what doesn't, and we've boiled down our findings to the five most impactful steps you can take to improve your performance on the test. We start at the beginning with study planning and move through the preparation process, all the way to the testing strategies that will help you get the most out of what you know when you're finally sitting in front of the test.

We recommend that you start preparing for your test as far in advance as possible. However, if you've bought this guide as a last-minute study resource and only have a few days before your test, we recommend that you skip over the first two Secret Keys since they address a long-term study plan.

If you struggle with **test anxiety**, we strongly encourage you to check out our recommendations for how you can overcome it. Test anxiety is a formidable foe, but it can be beaten, and we want to make sure you have the tools you need to defeat it.

Secret Key #1 – Plan Big, Study Small

There's a lot riding on your performance. If you want to ace this test, you're going to need to keep your skills sharp and the material fresh in your mind. You need a plan that lets you review everything you need to know while still fitting in your schedule. We'll break this strategy down into three categories.

Information Organization

Start with the information you already have: the official test outline. From this, you can make a complete list of all the concepts you need to cover before the test. Organize these concepts into groups that can be studied together, and create a list of any related vocabulary you need to learn so you can brush up on any difficult terms. You'll want to keep this vocabulary list handy once you actually start studying since you may need to add to it along the way.

Time Management

Once you have your set of study concepts, decide how to spread them out over the time you have left before the test. Break your study plan into small, clear goals so you have a manageable task for each day and know exactly what you're doing. Then just focus on one small step at a time. When you manage your time this way, you don't need to spend hours at a time studying. Studying a small block of content for a short period each day helps you retain information better and avoid stressing over how much you have left to do. You can relax knowing that you have a plan to cover everything in time. In order for this strategy to be effective though, you have to start studying early and stick to your schedule. Avoid the exhaustion and futility that comes from last-minute cramming!

Study Environment

The environment you study in has a big impact on your learning. Studying in a coffee shop, while probably more enjoyable, is not likely to be as fruitful as studying in a quiet room. It's important to keep distractions to a minimum. You're only planning to study for a short block of time, so make the most of it. Don't pause to check your phone or get up to find a snack. It's also important to **avoid multitasking**. Research has consistently shown that multitasking will make your studying dramatically less effective. Your study area should also be comfortable and well-lit so you don't have the distraction of straining your eyes or sitting on an uncomfortable chair.

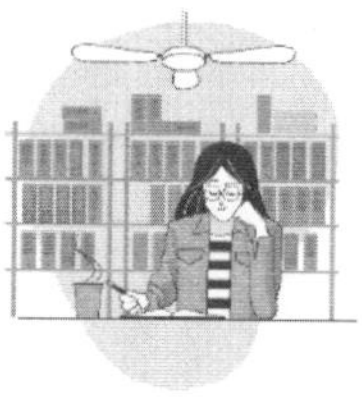

The time of day you study is also important. You want to be rested and alert. Don't wait until just before bedtime. Study when you'll be most likely to comprehend and remember. Even better, if you know what time of day your test will be, set that time aside for study. That way your brain will be used to working on that subject at that specific time and you'll have a better chance of recalling information.

Finally, it can be helpful to team up with others who are studying for the same test. Your actual studying should be done in as isolated an environment as possible, but the work of organizing the information and setting up the study plan can be divided up. In between study sessions, you can discuss with your teammates the concepts that you're all studying and quiz each other on the details. Just be sure that your teammates are as serious about the test as you are. If you find that your study time is being replaced with social time, you might need to find a new team.

Secret Key #2 – Make Your Studying Count

You're devoting a lot of time and effort to preparing for this test, so you want to be absolutely certain it will pay off. This means doing more than just reading the content and hoping you can remember it on test day. It's important to make every minute of study count. There are two main areas you can focus on to make your studying count.

Retention

It doesn't matter how much time you study if you can't remember the material. You need to make sure you are retaining the concepts. To check your retention of the information you're learning, try recalling it at later times with minimal prompting. Try carrying around flashcards and glance at one or two from time to time or ask a friend who's also studying for the test to quiz you.

To enhance your retention, look for ways to put the information into practice so that you can apply it rather than simply recalling it. If you're using the information in practical ways, it will be much easier to remember. Similarly, it helps to solidify a concept in your mind if you're not only reading it to yourself but also explaining it to someone else. Ask a friend to let you teach them about a concept you're a little shaky on (or speak aloud to an imaginary audience if necessary). As you try to summarize, define, give examples, and answer your friend's questions, you'll understand the concepts better and they will stay with you longer. Finally, step back for a big picture view and ask yourself how each piece of information fits with the whole subject. When you link the different concepts together and see them working together as a whole, it's easier to remember the individual components.

Finally, practice showing your work on any multi-step problems, even if you're just studying. Writing out each step you take to solve a problem will help solidify the process in your mind, and you'll be more likely to remember it during the test.

Modality

Modality simply refers to the means or method by which you study. Choosing a study modality that fits your own individual learning style is crucial. No two people learn best in exactly the same way, so it's important to know your strengths and use them to your advantage.

For example, if you learn best by visualization, focus on visualizing a concept in your mind and draw an image or a diagram. Try color-coding your notes, illustrating them, or creating symbols that will trigger your mind to recall a learned concept. If you learn best by hearing or discussing information, find a study partner who learns the same way or read aloud to yourself. Think about how to put the information in your own words. Imagine that you are giving a lecture on the topic and record yourself so you can listen to it later.

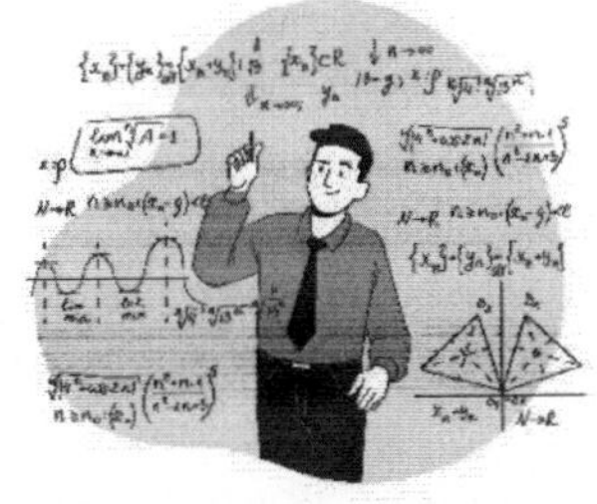

For any learning style, flashcards can be helpful. Organize the information so you can take advantage of spare moments to review. Underline key words or phrases. Use different colors for different categories. Mnemonic devices (such as creating a short list in which every item starts with the same letter) can also help with retention. Find what works best for you and use it to store the information in your mind most effectively and easily.

Secret Key #3 – Practice the Right Way

Your success on test day depends not only on how many hours you put into preparing, but also on whether you prepared the right way. It's good to check along the way to see if your studying is paying off. One of the most effective ways to do this is by taking practice tests to evaluate your progress. Practice tests are useful because they show exactly where you need to improve. Every time you take a practice test, pay special attention to these three groups of questions:

- The questions you got wrong
- The questions you had to guess on, even if you guessed right
- The questions you found difficult or slow to work through

This will show you exactly what your weak areas are, and where you need to devote more study time. Ask yourself why each of these questions gave you trouble. Was it because you didn't understand the material? Was it because you didn't remember the vocabulary? Do you need more repetitions on this type of question to build speed and confidence? Dig into those questions and figure out how you can strengthen your weak areas as you go back to review the material.

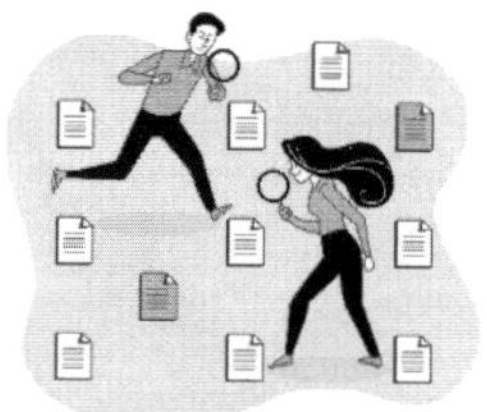

Additionally, many practice tests have a section explaining the answer choices. It can be tempting to read the explanation and think that you now have a good understanding of the concept. However, an explanation likely only covers part of the question's broader context. Even if the explanation makes perfect sense, **go back and investigate** every concept related to the question until you're positive you have a thorough understanding.

As you go along, keep in mind that the practice test is just that: practice. Memorizing these questions and answers will not be very helpful on the actual test because it is unlikely to have any of the same exact questions. If you only know the right answers to the sample questions, you won't be prepared for the real thing. **Study the concepts** until you understand them fully, and then you'll be able to answer any question that shows up on the test.

It's important to wait on the practice tests until you're ready. If you take a test on your first day of study, you may be overwhelmed by the amount of material covered and how much you need to learn. Work up to it gradually.

On test day, you'll need to be prepared for answering questions, managing your time, and using the test-taking strategies you've learned. It's a lot to balance, like a mental marathon that will have a big impact on your future. Like training for a marathon, you'll need to start slowly and work your way up. When test day arrives, you'll be ready.

Start with the strategies you've read in the first two Secret Keys—plan your course and study in the way that works best for you. If you have time, consider using multiple study resources to get different approaches to the same concepts. It can be helpful to see difficult concepts from more than one angle. Then find a good source for practice tests. Many times, the test website will suggest potential study resources or provide sample tests.

Practice Test Strategy

If you're able to find at least three practice tests, we recommend this strategy:

Untimed and Open-Book Practice

Take the first test with no time constraints and with your notes and study guide handy. Take your time and focus on applying the strategies you've learned.

Timed and Open-Book Practice

Take the second practice test open-book as well, but set a timer and practice pacing yourself to finish in time.

Timed and Closed-Book Practice

Take any other practice tests as if it were test day. Set a timer and put away your study materials. Sit at a table or desk in a quiet room, imagine yourself at the testing center, and answer questions as quickly and accurately as possible.

Keep repeating timed and closed-book tests on a regular basis until you run out of practice tests or it's time for the actual test. Your mind will be ready for the schedule and stress of test day, and you'll be able to focus on recalling the material you've learned.

Secret Key #4 – Pace Yourself

Once you're fully prepared for the material on the test, your biggest challenge on test day will be managing your time. Just knowing that the clock is ticking can make you panic even if you have plenty of time left. Work on pacing yourself so you can build confidence against the time constraints of the exam. Pacing is a difficult skill to master, especially in a high-pressure environment, so **practice is vital**.

Set time expectations for your pace based on how much time is available. For example, if a section has 60 questions and the time limit is 30 minutes, you know you have to average 30 seconds or less per question in order to answer them all. Although 30 seconds is the hard limit, set 25 seconds per question as your goal, so you reserve extra time to spend on harder questions. When you budget extra time for the harder questions, you no longer have any reason to stress when those questions take longer to answer.

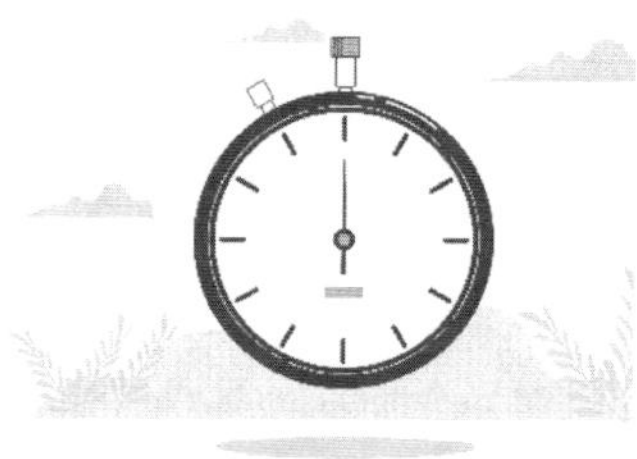

Don't let this time expectation distract you from working through the test at a calm, steady pace, but keep it in mind so you don't spend too much time on any one question. Recognize that taking extra time on one question you don't understand may keep you from answering two that you do understand later in the test. If your time limit for a question is up and you're still not sure of the answer, mark it and move on, and come back to it later if the time and the test format allow. If the testing format doesn't allow you to return to earlier questions, just make an educated guess; then put it out of your mind and move on.

On the easier questions, be careful not to rush. It may seem wise to hurry through them so you have more time for the challenging ones, but it's not worth missing one if you know the concept and just didn't take the time to read the question fully. Work efficiently but make sure you understand the question and have looked at all of the answer choices, since more than one may seem right at first.

Even if you're paying attention to the time, you may find yourself a little behind at some point. You should speed up to get back on track, but do so wisely. Don't panic; just take a few seconds less on each question until you're caught up. Don't guess without thinking, but do look through the answer choices and eliminate any you know are wrong. If you can get down to two choices, it is often worthwhile to guess from those. Once you've chosen an answer, move on and don't dwell on any that you skipped or had to hurry through. If a question was taking too long, chances are it was one of the harder ones, so you weren't as likely to get it right anyway.

On the other hand, if you find yourself getting ahead of schedule, it may be beneficial to slow down a little. The more quickly you work, the more likely you are to make a careless mistake that will affect your score. You've budgeted time for each question, so don't be afraid to spend that time. Practice an efficient but careful pace to get the most out of the time you have.

Secret Key #5 – Have a Plan for Guessing

When you're taking the test, you may find yourself stuck on a question. Some of the answer choices seem better than others, but you don't see the one answer choice that is obviously correct. What do you do?

The scenario described above is very common, yet most test takers have not effectively prepared for it. Developing and practicing a plan for guessing may be one of the single most effective uses of your time as you get ready for the exam.

In developing your plan for guessing, there are three questions to address:

- When should you start the guessing process?
- How should you narrow down the choices?
- Which answer should you choose?

When to Start the Guessing Process

Unless your plan for guessing is to select C every time (which, despite its merits, is not what we recommend), you need to leave yourself enough time to apply your answer elimination strategies. Since you have a limited amount of time for each question, that means that if you're going to give yourself the best shot at guessing correctly, you have to decide quickly whether or not you will guess.

Of course, the best-case scenario is that you don't have to guess at all, so first, see if you can answer the question based on your knowledge of the subject and basic reasoning skills. Focus on the key words in the question and try to jog your memory of related topics. Give yourself a chance to bring the knowledge to mind, but once you realize that you don't have (or you can't access) the knowledge you need to answer the question, it's time to start the guessing process.

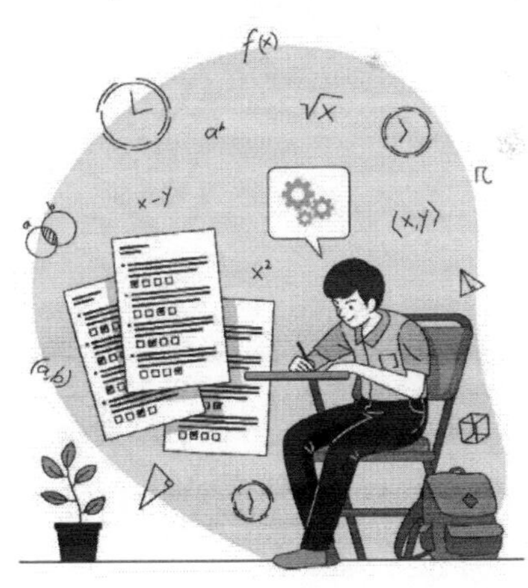

It's almost always better to start the guessing process too early than too late. It only takes a few seconds to remember something and answer the question from knowledge. Carefully eliminating wrong answer choices takes longer. Plus, going through the process of eliminating answer choices can actually help jog your memory.

Summary: Start the guessing process as soon as you decide that you can't answer the question based on your knowledge.

How to Narrow Down the Choices

The next chapter in this book (**Test-Taking Strategies**) includes a wide range of strategies for how to approach questions and how to look for answer choices to eliminate. You will definitely want to read those carefully, practice them, and figure out which ones work best for you. Here though, we're going to address a mindset rather than a particular strategy.

Your odds of guessing an answer correctly depend on how many options you are choosing from.

Number of options left	5	4	3	2	1
Odds of guessing correctly	20%	25%	33%	50%	100%

You can see from this chart just how valuable it is to be able to eliminate incorrect answers and make an educated guess, but there are two things that many test takers do that cause them to miss out on the benefits of guessing:

- Accidentally eliminating the correct answer
- Selecting an answer based on an impression

We'll look at the first one here, and the second one in the next section.

To avoid accidentally eliminating the correct answer, we recommend a thought exercise called **the $5 challenge**. In this challenge, you only eliminate an answer choice from contention if you are willing to bet $5 on it being wrong. Why $5? Five dollars is a small but not insignificant amount of money. It's an amount you could afford to lose but wouldn't want to throw away. And while losing $5 once might not hurt too much, doing it twenty times will set you back $100. In the same way, each small decision you make—eliminating a choice here, guessing on a question there—won't by itself impact your score very much, but when you put them all together, they can make a big difference. By holding each answer choice elimination decision to a higher standard, you can reduce the risk of accidentally eliminating the correct answer.

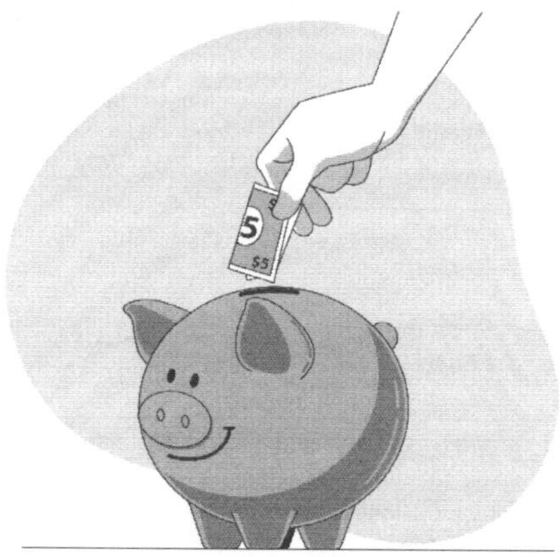

The $5 challenge can also be applied in a positive sense: If you are willing to bet $5 that an answer choice *is* correct, go ahead and mark it as correct.

Summary: Only eliminate an answer choice if you are willing to bet $5 that it is wrong.

Which Answer to Choose

You're taking the test. You've run into a hard question and decided you'll have to guess. You've eliminated all the answer choices you're willing to bet $5 on. Now you have to pick an answer. Why do we even need to talk about this? Why can't you just pick whichever one you feel like when the time comes?

The answer to these questions is that if you don't come into the test with a plan, you'll rely on your impression to select an answer choice, and if you do that, you risk falling into a trap. The test writers know that everyone who takes their test will be guessing on some of the questions, so they intentionally write wrong answer choices to seem plausible. You still have to pick an answer though, and if the wrong answer choices are designed to look right, how can you ever be sure that you're not falling for their trap? The best solution we've found to this dilemma is to take the decision out of your hands entirely. Here is the process we recommend:

Once you've eliminated any choices that you are confident (willing to bet $5) are wrong, select the first remaining choice as your answer.

Whether you choose to select the first remaining choice, the second, or the last, the important thing is that you use some preselected standard. Using this approach guarantees that you will not be enticed into selecting an answer choice that looks right, because you are not basing your decision on how the answer choices look.

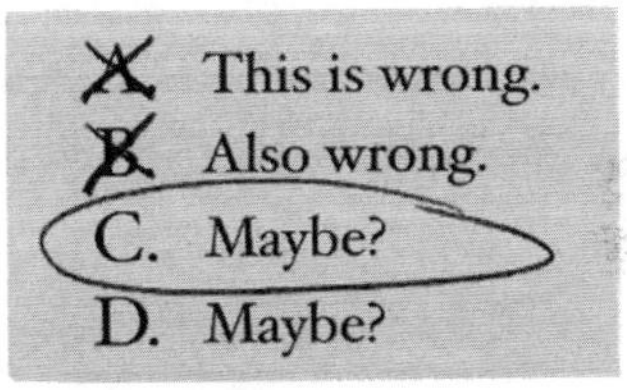

This is not meant to make you question your knowledge. Instead, it is to help you recognize the difference between your knowledge and your impressions. There's a huge difference between thinking an answer is right because of what you know, and thinking an answer is right because it looks or sounds like it should be right.

Summary: To ensure that your selection is appropriately random, make a predetermined selection from among all answer choices you have not eliminated.

Test-Taking Strategies

This section contains a list of test-taking strategies that you may find helpful as you work through the test. By taking what you know and applying logical thought, you can maximize your chances of answering any question correctly!

It is very important to realize that every question is different and every person is different: no single strategy will work on every question, and no single strategy will work for every person. That's why we've included all of them here, so you can try them out and determine which ones work best for different types of questions and which ones work best for you.

Question Strategies

☑ Read Carefully

Read the question and the answer choices carefully. Don't miss the question because you misread the terms. You have plenty of time to read each question thoroughly and make sure you understand what is being asked. Yet a happy medium must be attained, so don't waste too much time. You must read carefully and efficiently.

☑ Contextual Clues

Look for contextual clues. If the question includes a word you are not familiar with, look at the immediate context for some indication of what the word might mean. Contextual clues can often give you all the information you need to decipher the meaning of an unfamiliar word. Even if you can't determine the meaning, you may be able to narrow down the possibilities enough to make a solid guess at the answer to the question.

☑ Prefixes

If you're having trouble with a word in the question or answer choices, try dissecting it. Take advantage of every clue that the word might include. Prefixes can be a huge help. Usually, they allow you to determine a basic meaning. *Pre-* means before, *post-* means after, *pro-* is positive, *de-* is negative. From prefixes, you can get an idea of the general meaning of the word and try to put it into context.

☑ Hedge Words

Watch out for critical hedge words, such as *likely, may, can, often, almost, mostly, usually, generally, rarely,* and *sometimes.* Question writers insert these hedge phrases to cover every possibility. Often an answer choice will be wrong simply because it leaves no room for exception. Be on guard for answer choices that have definitive words such as *exactly* and *always.*

☑ Switchback Words

Stay alert for *switchbacks.* These are the words and phrases frequently used to alert you to shifts in thought. The most common switchback words are *but, although,* and *however.* Others include *nevertheless, on the other hand, even though, while, in spite of, despite,* and *regardless of.* Switchback words are important to catch because they can change the direction of the question or an answer choice.

⊘ Face Value

When in doubt, use common sense. Accept the situation in the problem at face value. Don't read too much into it. These problems will not require you to make wild assumptions. If you have to go beyond creativity and warp time or space in order to have an answer choice fit the question, then you should move on and consider the other answer choices. These are normal problems rooted in reality. The applicable relationship or explanation may not be readily apparent, but it is there for you to figure out. Use your common sense to interpret anything that isn't clear.

Answer Choice Strategies

⊘ Answer Selection

The most thorough way to pick an answer choice is to identify and eliminate wrong answers until only one is left, then confirm it is the correct answer. Sometimes an answer choice may immediately seem right, but be careful. The test writers will usually put more than one reasonable answer choice on each question, so take a second to read all of them and make sure that the other choices are not equally obvious. As long as you have time left, it is better to read every answer choice than to pick the first one that looks right without checking the others.

⊘ Answer Choice Families

An answer choice family consists of two (in rare cases, three) answer choices that are very similar in construction and cannot all be true at the same time. If you see two answer choices that are direct opposites or parallels, one of them is usually the correct answer. For instance, if one answer choice says that quantity *x* increases and another either says that quantity *x* decreases (opposite) or says that quantity *y* increases (parallel), then those answer choices would fall into the same family. An answer choice that doesn't match the construction of the answer choice family is more likely to be incorrect. Most questions will not have answer choice families, but when they do appear, you should be prepared to recognize them.

⊘ Eliminate Answers

Eliminate answer choices as soon as you realize they are wrong, but make sure you consider all possibilities. If you are eliminating answer choices and realize that the last one you are left with is also wrong, don't panic. Start over and consider each choice again. There may be something you missed the first time that you will realize on the second pass.

⊘ Avoid Fact Traps

Don't be distracted by an answer choice that is factually true but doesn't answer the question. You are looking for the choice that answers the question. Stay focused on what the question is asking for so you don't accidentally pick an answer that is true but incorrect. Always go back to the question and make sure the answer choice you've selected actually answers the question and is not merely a true statement.

⊘ Extreme Statements

In general, you should avoid answers that put forth extreme actions as standard practice or proclaim controversial ideas as established fact. An answer choice that states the "process should be used in certain situations, if..." is much more likely to be correct than one that states the "process should be discontinued completely." The first is a calm rational statement and doesn't even make a definitive, uncompromising stance, using a hedge word *if* to provide wiggle room, whereas the second choice is far more extreme.

⊘ Benchmark

As you read through the answer choices and you come across one that seems to answer the question well, mentally select that answer choice. This is not your final answer, but it's the one that will help you evaluate the other answer choices. The one that you selected is your benchmark or standard for judging each of the other answer choices. Every other answer choice must be compared to your benchmark. That choice is correct until proven otherwise by another answer choice beating it. If you find a better answer, then that one becomes your new benchmark. Once you've decided that no other choice answers the question as well as your benchmark, you have your final answer.

⊘ Predict the Answer

Before you even start looking at the answer choices, it is often best to try to predict the answer. When you come up with the answer on your own, it is easier to avoid distractions and traps because you will know exactly what to look for. The right answer choice is unlikely to be word-for-word what you came up with, but it should be a close match. Even if you are confident that you have the right answer, you should still take the time to read each option before moving on.

General Strategies

⊘ Tough Questions

If you are stumped on a problem or it appears too hard or too difficult, don't waste time. Move on! Remember though, if you can quickly check for obviously incorrect answer choices, your chances of guessing correctly are greatly improved. Before you completely give up, at least try to knock out a couple of possible answers. Eliminate what you can and then guess at the remaining answer choices before moving on.

⊘ Check Your Work

Since you will probably not know every term listed and the answer to every question, it is important that you get credit for the ones that you do know. Don't miss any questions through careless mistakes. If at all possible, try to take a second to look back over your answer selection and make sure you've selected the correct answer choice and haven't made a costly careless mistake (such as marking an answer choice that you didn't mean to mark). This quick double check should more than pay for itself in caught mistakes for the time it costs.

⊘ Pace Yourself

It's easy to be overwhelmed when you're looking at a page full of questions; your mind is confused and full of random thoughts, and the clock is ticking down faster than you would like. Calm down and maintain the pace that you have set for yourself. Especially as you get down to the last few minutes of the test, don't let the small numbers on the clock make you panic. As long as you are on track by monitoring your pace, you are guaranteed to have time for each question.

⊘ Don't Rush

It is very easy to make errors when you are in a hurry. Maintaining a fast pace in answering questions is pointless if it makes you miss questions that you would have gotten right otherwise. Test writers like to include distracting information and wrong answers that seem right. Taking a little extra time to avoid careless mistakes can make all the difference in your test score. Find a pace that allows you to be confident in the answers that you select.

☑ Keep Moving

Panicking will not help you pass the test, so do your best to stay calm and keep moving. Taking deep breaths and going through the answer elimination steps you practiced can help to break through a stress barrier and keep your pace.

Final Notes

The combination of a solid foundation of content knowledge and the confidence that comes from practicing your plan for applying that knowledge is the key to maximizing your performance on test day. As your foundation of content knowledge is built up and strengthened, you'll find that the strategies included in this chapter become more and more effective in helping you quickly sift through the distractions and traps of the test to isolate the correct answer.

Now that you're preparing to move forward into the test content chapters of this book, be sure to keep your goal in mind. As you read, think about how you will be able to apply this information on the test. If you've already seen sample questions for the test and you have an idea of the question format and style, try to come up with questions of your own that you can answer based on what you're reading. This will give you valuable practice applying your knowledge in the same ways you can expect to on test day.

Good luck and good studying!

Patient Education and Assessment

Breast Cancer

Routine examination of the breast should enable the identification of early changes that indicate underlying pathology and then allow intervention before such changes become life threatening. The American Cancer Society recommends monthly breast self-examination beginning at age 20 and clinical breast examination every three years from age 20 to 39 and annually thereafter. They recommend an annual mammogram after age 40 with no upper age limit. Other guidelines suggest that, after a baseline mammogram at age 40, further mammograms may be performed every 1 or 2 years until age 50, depending on the history and clinical findings of the individual woman.

Breast cancer is the second most common malignancy in American women (after non-melanoma skin cancer) and the second leading cause of cancer death in women (after lung cancer). One in eight women in the United States will be diagnosed with breast cancer during her lifetime and one in thirty-three will die from it. The American Cancer Society reports that approximately 213,000 women in the United States are diagnosed with invasive breast cancer each year – this produced an incidence rate of 100.6 cases per 100,000 women during the 1990's. Less than 0.5% of breast cancers occur in women under 30, 3.5% from age 30-39, 19% from age 40-49, and 77% in women over 50. Only 1% of breast cancers occur in men where the incidence rate is 1 per 100,000.

Breast Self-Examination

Breast self-examination should be done monthly after age 20. It should be performed one week after the menstrual period when there is no tenderness or swelling or, in non-menstruating women, on the same day each month. This requires proper instruction and periodic review in order to enable a woman to become familiar with the composition of her breasts and to recognize changes. She starts by moving her hand gently over the skin of each breast, right hand on left breast and left hand on right breast, checking for lumps and thickening. This step is most easily done in the shower when the skin is wet and without resistance. Next she stands in front of a mirror, first with hands at her sides and then with arms raised. She looks for changes in shape, swelling, skin color or thickness and nipple changes. She then places her hands on her hips to flex the chest muscles and looks for the same changes. Finally she lies down with a pillow under her right shoulder and her right arm behind her head. With the pads of three fingers on her left hand she makes small circular motions in a pattern that will cover the entire surface of her right breast. Alternative patterns include vertical lines following an imaginary grid and a wedge pattern starting at the outer edges and ending at the nipple. She squeezes the nipple to check for discharges or lumps and then follows the same steps with the right hand on the left breast.

Risk Factors

Women at a higher risk of developing breast cancer should have more frequent mammograms. These risk factors include: changes on clinical breast examination, a prior diagnosis of breast or any other cancer, a previous biopsy read as lobular neoplasia or atypical hyperplasia, two or more previous biopsies regardless of the reading, a known mutation in a cancer susceptibility gene (BRAC1 or BRAC2), a primary female relative (mother, sister, or daughter) with a diagnosis of breast cancer, or age over 40 with at least 75% breast density. Continuous exposure of the breast to estrogen (endogenous or exogenous) as in early menarche, late menopause, late age of birth of first child, never having been pregnant, and prolonged use of oral contraceptives or hormone replacement therapy, are also considered risk factors.

Historical risk factors include a previous diagnosis of breast or any other cancer in the patient or blood relatives, age over 50, and endogenous or exogenous estrogen exposure. Clinical findings of breast pain or tenderness, lumps or swelling not previously noted, skin hardening or thickening, nipple discharge (red or red-brown is of more concern than clear, milky, yellow, or green), rash-like changes on the skin, areolae, or nipples, nipple flattening or inversion, or swelling, redness, dimpling, or puckering of the skin would indicate that further workup for potential breast pathology is indicated.

Clinical Breast Examination

A clinical breast examination by a health care professional should be done every three years from age 20 to 39 and annually thereafter. This requires training and consistent practice on the part of the clinician. First observe the woman sitting to compare size and shape of the breasts and look for bulges and retractions. Look for swelling or redness of the skin and symmetry or changes in the nipples. Make the same observations with the woman standing with her hands at her sides, over head, and when pressing her hands against her hips to flex the chest muscles. While she is still standing, palpate the axillary and supraclavicular lymph nodes and gently palpate the breasts without pinching the tissue between the fingers. Use a predetermined pattern that will cover each breast in its entirety. Repeat the palpation on both sides with the woman lying down with the arm on that side raised above her head.

Breast Ultrasound

In ultrasound examination of the breast, high frequency sound waves are bounced off surfaces within the breast, reflected back, and converted to video or photographic images. The technique is not FDA approved as a screening tool in asymptomatic women because of poor resolution of these images. Ultrasound is non-invasive and useful in women with dense breasts, women who should not be exposed to X-rays (e.g. pregnant women,) and women with silicone implants. It is helpful in lesions not classified by mammography and particularly useful in distinguishing fluid-filled cysts from solid masses. Ultrasound is also useful in guiding needle biopsy.

Mammography

Mammography is an X-ray examination that is used as a screening tool in asymptomatic women. Some malignancies may be seen by mammography two years before they are large enough to be felt by examination, so an annual mammogram is recommended for women over 40. X-rays are differentially absorbed by various tissues. They are least discriminating in women with dense breasts and highly discriminating for small calcium deposits. The technique is not tissue specific and cannot differentiate benign from malignant lesions by absorption alone. A trained practitioner must interpret mammograms, and audits of individual practice help establish reliability and validity of these interpretations. X-rays are recorded on screen-film cassettes or by electronic digital imaging. In computer-assisted detection, the computer is programmed to flag what might be an abnormality. This still requires interpretation by a radiologist. Mammography is non-invasive, relatively inexpensive, and standardized so that annual images may be compared with prior ones. The X-ray dose is usually limited to 0.1 – 0.2 rads per view.

Ductography

For a breast ductogram, a hair-sized needle or tube is threaded into a single discharging nipple duct and a small amount of iodinated contrast material is injected. On a magnified view during mammography, one can then identify filling defects, obstructions, and cysts. Tissue may also be obtained for cytological examination. Multiple discharging ducts are not an indication for this procedure. The ductogram may serve as a guide for surgery. Ductography is contraindicated in women who are allergic to the contrast material.

MRI

Magnetic resonance imaging (MRI) uses a strong magnetic field and pulses of radio wave energy to provide an image. It is not a screening tool and is used when questions are raised by mammography or ultrasound, particularly in women with dense breasts. It is most useful in examining tissue close to the chest wall and, with contrast material in the blood, to show tumors with increased vascularization. It helps pre-operatively to show the extent of these tumors and post-operatively to see residual tumor or reoccurrence. MRIs cannot show microcalcifications. This is an expensive, in-hospital procedure that is contraindicated when there is metal (e.g. a pacemaker) in the body, a woman is pregnant or allergic to contrast material, or a woman is anxious in closed spaces, unable to like face down and be completely still for up to two hours, or too overweight to fit in the machine.

Sentinel Node Mapping

It is hypothesized that a specific lymph channel may drain a primary tumor and lead to a first or "sentinel" node in that primary drainage area. Usually there are 1 to 3 "sentinel" nodes. The drainage pattern may be demonstrated visually with a blue dye or with technetium 99, a low level radioactive tracer, using a hand-held Geiger counter over the skin. With this technique, the surgeon can determine if the tumor goes beyond the first node and further dissection is necessary. The procedure produces less pain and fewer complications than a full axillary dissection because no drains are inserted.

Pneumocystography

If a cyst is demonstrated on mammography or ultrasound, then a needle can be inserted into it and fluid withdrawn for cytological examination. Air can then be injected in order to visualize the wall of the cyst. Obvious tumors can then be biopsied. The procedure itself may be therapeutic if the cyst does not reoccur after the air injection. Surgical removal of benign cysts may also be avoided. The procedure itself can be painful.

Biopsy Techniques

In **fine needle aspiration**, the needle is advanced and withdrawn multiple times within the mass. Material from within the needle is smeared onto a slide. While the technique is simple, safe, accurate, well tolerated, inexpensive, and requires no special equipment, the interpretation of such small fragments requires a skilled cytopathologist.

A **core needle biopsy** is done with a special spring-loaded needle that is fired into the mass and a core sample removed. This better sample improves histological interpretation, but requires a preliminary incision through the skin under local anesthesia.

An **excisional biopsy** removes the whole mass. This requires local or general anesthesia and surgical closure. The entire sample may be examined and the margins examined for abnormal cells.

Simple Mastectomy

In a simple mastectomy the breast with skin and nipple intact is removed but lymph nodes are not dissected. There may be a separate incision for sentinel node biopsy. With this procedure there is less chance for local recurrence than with a lumpectomy. Reconstruction may be done as part of the same procedure. Possible complications of the procedure include wound infection, blood or fluid in the wound, lymphedema if nodes are removed, numbness in the upper arm, and phantom breast pain.

Lumpectomy

In a lumpectomy (known as "breast conserving therapy" in Europe) only the tumor tissue and surrounding tissue to clean margins on histological examination is removed. Examination of frozen sections from the operating room must be considered preliminary, and, if malignant cells are found at the margin on fixed specimens, then return for further surgery may be indicated. The procedure is indicated if there is no evidence of tumor in other sites on mammography, the patient is younger and has no genetic markers for breast cancer. Concern for cosmetic appearance, body image, and the feeling of sexual desirability may also be considered. Lumpectomy is contraindicated when there has been previous radiation treatment of the breast, a previous lumpectomy, multiple tumors in the breast, connective tissue disease, a tumor over 2" in diameter, or a large tumor in a small breast.

Lumpectomy removes only the tumor tissue and the surrounding tissue to margins that are clean on histological examination. Radiation, either intraoperative or postoperative, is used to treat microscopic invasion. A second incision in the axilla allows for dissection of lymph nodes. This may be either a "sentinel" node biopsy or more extensive dissection where multiple nodes are sent for histological examination. Side effects of radiation may include localized hair loss, fatigue, skin rash or redness, decreased appetite, and increased nausea. Side effects of axillary dissection include lymphedema or swelling of the arm, limitation of arm and shoulder movement, and numbness of the skin on the upper arm.

Radiation Therapy

Radiation is used as a non-surgical alternative or adjunct to surgery for breast or any other cancer because it is toxic to rapidly proliferating cells. Malignant cells proliferate rapidly, but so do cells in bone marrow, buccal and intestinal mucosa, hair follicles, and the urinary bladder. Radiation is targeted to tumor cells, however, so that other rapidly proliferating cells may be spared. An external beam may be directed at the affected area of the breast. This is usually done five times per week for six weeks on an outpatient basis. The most common side effects are general fatigue, loss of appetite, "sunburn" of the skin, and breast swelling and tenderness. With internal radiation, tiny tubes are implanted near the tumor and pellets of radioactive Iridium-192 are placed in them seven times over the course of a week. This generally results in fewer and milder side effects than with external radiation.

Chemotherapy

The pharmacologic basis for the chemotherapeutic treatment of breast or any form of cancer is that some drugs interfere with the DNA synthesis, repair, and replication of rapidly proliferating cells. These drugs may be used to shrink tumors prior to surgery or be used in addition to or instead of surgery. Malignant cells proliferate rapidly, but so do cells in bone marrow, buccal and intestinal mucosa, hair follicles, and the urinary bladder. All of these cells are also affected by cancer chemotherapy so that common side effects include leucopenia (and subsequent infection), anemia, low platelet count, stomatitis, nausea and vomiting, gastrointestinal distress, hair loss, and urinary distress. Other potential hazards are birth defects, infertility, and early menopause. Side effects are usually dose and time related so that combination therapy using smaller doses of two drugs may reduce the side effects. Side effects may also respond to specific medications, e.g. antinausea drugs.

Hormone Therapy

More than half of breast tumors are sensitive to estrogen and so-called selective estrogen receptor modulators (SERM) bind to estrogen receptor sites and block the effect of estrogen on those tumors. One non-steroidal anti-estrogen, Tamoxifen, has been used for years to decrease the incidence of contralateral breast cancer after the first tumor has been excised. It promotes early menopause so cannot be used if pregnancy is anticipated. Low estrogen after menopause is also associated with loss of bone mineral density and osteoporosis. The use of Tamoxifen for prophylaxis in women at high risk of developing breast cancer (e.g. with genetic markers) is controversial because of a small incidence of uterine cancer, blood clots, and strokes associated with its use. With a newer non-steroidal anti-estrogen, raloxifene, there is less loss of bone mineral density. It may actually prevent osteoporosis in post-menopausal women.

Modified Radical Mastectomy

In a modified radical mastectomy the breast with skin and nipple intact and the axillary lymph nodes are removed. (A radical mastectomy where the underlying chest muscle is also removed is rarely done today.) Because of the lymph node dissection, drainage tubes are often left in for up to two weeks. Possible complications of the procedure include wound infection, blood or fluid in the wound, lymphedema, numbness in the upper arm, and phantom breast pain.

Breast Reconstruction

Breast implants usually consist of a silicone rubber shell filled with silicone gel, saline, or an alternative substance such as purified vegetable oil. They may be filled by the manufacturer or be adjusted either at the time of implantation or later. Saline implants are generally firmer and hold their shape better. They are FDA approved and the most common implants in use. Silicone gel implants are initially softer and feel more natural, but, over time, may develop capsular contraction and become hard. Concerns about implant leakage, silicone migration, and associated connective tissue disease have now dissipated and silicone implants are again FDA approved. Alternate substance implants are still considered investigational. Implants may be subglandular or submuscular and either placed at the time of reconstruction, or an expander placed at that time and the implant inserted 4 to 6 months later. It should not be assumed that implants will last a lifetime, and local complications such as breast pain, capsular contraction, change in sensation, or rupture often require a subsequent operation.

The **latissimus dorsi flap** is a pedicle flap of latissimus muscle, fatty tissue, and skin that is tunneled under the skin from the back to the reconstruction site on the breast. Preserving all the fatty tissue beneath Scarpa's fascia results in a more natural teardrop shape to the reconstructed breast. Large breasts may require an additional implant under the pectoralis muscle. This major operative procedure leaves scars on both the back and on the breast, but may be done on both sides of the body if necessary. In general, surgical flaps are contraindicated in women who are very overweight, smoke, have had previous surgery at the flap site, or have circulatory problems. Very thin women may not have enough tissue to provide a flap.

The **transverse rectus abdominis myocutaneous (TRAM) flap** is a pedicle flap of rectus muscle, fatty tissue, and skin that is tunneled under the skin from the abdomen to the reconstruction site on the breast. Blood supply to the muscle is retained, but nerve connections are not. The flap may also be removed and reattached rather than tunneled. This major operative procedure leaves scars on both the abdomen and on the breast, could become problematic if the recipient becomes pregnant, and can be done only once. In general, surgical flaps are contraindicated in women who are very overweight, smoke, have had previous surgery at the flap site, or have circulatory problems. Very thin women may not have enough tissue to provide a flap.

Instrumentation and Quality Assurance

X-Ray Tubes

The **anode** targets most commonly used in mammography are molybdenum and rhodium because of their characteristic radiation energy. X-ray **filters** remove the low energy photons that increase patient dose without enhancing the image. Molybdenum is the most commonly used filter material in mammography. In order to meet federal regulations, any filter must be equivalent to a 0.5 mm aluminum standard. The material used in X-ray tube exit ports or **windows** is beryllium because, unlike glass, it does not attenuate the beam. The angle between the surface of the anode target and a vertical line perpendicular to the image receptor is called the anode angle. This result is what is called the anode heel effect or decreased output to the anode side of the field.

Kilovoltage Peak and Range

Kilovoltage peak (kVp) is the maximum value of the potential difference between the anode and cathode in an x-ray tube and determines the maximum energy of X-rays emitted by that tube. The range depends on the target/filtration element (molybdenum, rhodium, or tungsten). In thicker breasts, more radiation is needed because there is more absorption. Increasing kVp lowers the dose but reduces contrast. Decreasing kVp increases the dose but also increases contrast.

AEC

The automatic exposure control (AEC) is an X-ray sensor located below the image receptor and beneath the densest part of the breast. The AEC controls the length of exposure after there has been adequate x-ray penetration of the glandular tissue. Systems have at least three positions or multiple sensors to assure adequate penetration of the densest part of the breast.

Mammography Compression Devices

Compressing the breast creates a decreased and uniform breast thickness that allows for lower radiation dose and shorter exposure time while stabilizing the breast during the procedure. A flat-surface compression paddle parallel to the breast support has a perpendicular 2-4 cm wall at the patient side to keep unwanted skin and tissue out of the image. The American College of Radiology recommends that the paddle must not be more than 1 cm out of parallel with the breast support and must not extend more than 1% of the source-image-distance beyond the chest wall edge of the film. There should be both automatic and manual modes to apply 25 to 45 pounds (111 to 200 Newtons) of initial compression force that is then maintained until released. In case of power failure, there must be a way to manually release compression.

System Geometry

System geometry refers to the spatial relationship of the X-ray source, patient, and image receptor. The source-image-distance (SID) is the distance from the X-ray source to the image receptor and, the longer that distance, the lower the radiation exposure and the lower the magnification. The typical mammography SID is 60-65 cm but it can range from 55 to 76 cm. The object-image receptor-distance (OID) should be as small as possible except when magnification is needed. When the breast is elevated to reduce the source-object-distance (SOD), magnification increases. For a magnification factor of 2, the breast would be half way between the focal spot on the anode and the film.

Grids

Grids are used to decrease scattered radiation and thereby improve image contrast. The grid is placed below the breast support and above the film cassette. The grid consists of a series of thin strips (usually lead or tantalum) separated by interspace material such as wood or fiber. The grid ratio (height of strip over separation between strips) for mammography is 4-5:1 instead of the conventional 8-12:1. The frequency of these attenuation strips is usually 60-80 lines per cm. High transmission cellular (HTC) grids have crossed copper grid strips and air for interspace material. Grids remove both primary and scattered radiation and therefore increase the dose. The Bucky factor is the ratio of exposure with grid to that without grid. For mammography units, this is usually 2-3:1.

Intensifying Screens

The intensifying screen converts X-ray photons to light photons and reduces the amount of radiation required to expose film by 98-99% while improving **the** detail of the image. The screen is placed under the film with the emulsion side of the film in contact with the screen. The X-ray photon produces a scintillation or small point of light on the screen. This hits silver bromide crystals in the adjacent emulsion. To facilitate film-screen contact, all air must be allowed to bleed out before the film is exposed. This is generally referred to as the 15 minute "rest" between loading and exposing the film cassette.

Focal Spots

The focal spot is the area that electrons from the cathode strike on the anode target. Focal spot size refers to the area projected onto the patient. The smaller the target angle, the smaller the focal spot size. The large spot is used routinely in mammography and is generally 0.3 mm. The small spot (usually 0.1 mm) is used for magnification views in order to increase sharpness.

Film Processing

Some of the silver bromide crystals in the film emulsion are exposed to light in the X-ray process. In the developer solution, these are converted to silver metal that remains on the film to form the image. In the fixer solution, development stops and the unexposed crystals are washed out of the film. Washing removes chemical residue and drying then removes the water and allows the emulsion to harden. The mechanical subsystem determines the optimal rate of transit through the processor, and the replenishment subsystem maintains a consistent strength of chemicals.

The cassette facilitates screen-film contact without absorbing an undesirable amount of X-ray energy. Plastic cassettes absorb about 30% of X-rays and carbon-fiber ones about 15%. The cassette should be durable and allow no ambient light to penetrate. It allows placement of the film edge as close to the chest wall as possible. After film and screen are loaded into the cassette, the unit should be allowed to rest for 15 minutes until all the air bleeds out of it. Cassettes should be used in the order in which they are loaded.

"Characteristic Curves"

The characteristic curve (also known as the d-log-E or H&D curve) plots the relationship between the optical density of the film and its exposure. The lowest exposure is the reading recorded at the base of the curve, the useful range of optical densities fills the straight-line portion, and the highest level of exposure is recorded at the shoulder of the curve. From these curves, films may be compared with regard to base-plus-fog, speed, contrast, and maximum density for a simple exposure. The steeper the slope, the higher the contrast, and the faster the film, the more it shifts to the left of the scale.

Extended Processing

Extended processing uses a higher developer temperature and/or a longer development time for single-emulsion film. The advantages are that this allows for higher film speeds with lower exposure dose and provides higher contrast. The disadvantages are that it increases the risk of processing artifacts and an increase in film fog.

Digital Mammography

Digital technology utilizes an amorphous silicon-based flat panel detector and electronic system instead of film-screen. The image receptor plate consists of a protective layer, a phosphor layer, a conductive layer to conduct away static, a flexible support layer and a backing layer. Storage phosphors in the panel absorb X-rays and form a latent image. A computer reader scans the image with a laser beam to activate the storage phosphors to emit ultraviolet light. This light is collected and sent to a photo multiplier tube where it is then converted to a digital signal. This signal can be viewed, manipulated, and magnified at a workstation and then be printed, stored, or transmitted electronically.

Quality Control Tests

Pieces of lint, dust particles, or specks of dirt may create artifacts on film images; therefore, the darkroom must be cleaned thoroughly before the start of each workday. Food and drink are not allowed in the darkroom. The American College of Radiology recommends that nothing should be stored on open shelving above work surfaces and that unnecessary items should be removed from countertops and work surfaces. Stable relative humidity between 40% and 60% reduces the potential for static electricity that would attract particles. Air should be filtered coming into the darkroom. Procedurally, a clean, damp, lint-free towel should be used to wipe surfaces. The processor film tray should be cleaned last with an antistatic cleaning solution on a lint-free cloth; then the floor should then be damp mopped. The number of artifacts that appear on mammography images determines performance evaluation. Cleaning procedures should be documented and more frequent and/or thorough cleaning may be necessary if too many artifacts are visible.

Processor quality control: The film processor and processor chemistry must be tested before films are processed each day in order to assure that operating levels are consistent. Expose and process a sensitometric strip. Read and plot mid-density (MD), density difference (DD), and base-plus-fog (B+F) level on the control chart. The American College of Radiology states that MD must be within ± 0.15 of the established operating level, DD within ± 0.15 of established operating level, and B+F within + 0.03 of that established operating level. If the test falls outside these limits, then the source of the problem e.g. temperature, chemistry, or replenishment rate must be identified and corrected. Any significant change in chemicals, film, or monitoring devices requires a 5-day recalibration.

Operating levels: The film processor and processor chemistry must work in a consistent manner. This procedure will be carried out at the time of initial set-up or if there is a significant change in the process such as the introduction of a different brand of film or chemical or change in procedure or conditions. Testing requires a sensitometer, densitometer, box of control film, control chart and digital clinical thermometer accurate to

± 0.5° F. First drain all chemicals and wash all tanks and racks with water. Fill the developer and fixer tanks and their replenishment tanks with fresh solutions. Set the temperature and replenishment levels as specified by the manufacturer. Using a 21-step sensitometer, expose and process a sensitometric strip. Read and record the densities of each step with a densitometer. The American College of Radiology recommends that this be done for five consecutive days to determine which steps have average density closest to but not less than 1.20 (mid-density or MD), closest to 2.20 (high-density or HD), and closest to but not less that 0.45 (low-density or LD). The difference between HD and LD is density difference (DD). Then determine the density of an unexposed area on each of the five strips. This density is the base-plus-fog (B+F) level.

Screen cleanliness: Screens should be cleaned at least weekly so that they are free of any dirt or dust particles that would compromise the quality of the image or be mistaken for microcalcifications. Cleaning may be limited to dusting with a camel's hair brush or canned air. Cleaning with liquid screen cleaner should be done as needed and the screens then allowed to air dry. If white spots in the same location are noted on more than one mammogram, then the screen should be cleaned before subsequent films are made.

"Cross-over" film: Because there may be slight variations in each batch of radiographic film, a "cross-over" procedure is necessary before a new batch of film may be processed. For five days, sensitometric strips of both the old and new batches are exposed and processed. The average values for MD, DD, and B+F of both batches are determined and the old operating levels are adjusted accordingly.

Darkroom fog: Ambient light may fog mammography film, and this should be tested for every six months or when bulbs or filters are changed. Safelight filters, bulb wattage, and distance from safelight to film-handling surface should be in accord with the film manufacturer's instructions. First check for obvious light leaks. Then expose a phantom image under normal conditions. Remove the exposed film from the cassette and place it emulsion side up on the countertop. Cover half the film with an opaque card and leave it for two minutes. After the film is processed, determine the density difference between the covered and uncovered portions of the image. If the density difference exceeds 0.05, then the source of the light problem should be identified and corrected.

Compression: Adequate breast compression is essential for high quality images and the compression force is tested initially and every six months thereafter. A towel is placed on the cassette holder and a bathroom scale placed upon the towel. The scale should be of an analog type unless a digital scale specifically designed to measure compression force is used. More towels are placed on the scale to protect the compression device which is then lowered both automatically and manually until it stops. The compression force must be at least 111 newtons (25 pounds) but no more than 200 newtons (45 pounds). If these criteria are not met, then a qualified service engineer should make the appropriate adjustments.

Screen-film contact: Because of the higher resolution of mammography screen-film units, uniform contact is essential for the production of sharp images. Testing with 40 mesh (40 wires per inch) copper screen should be done when each cassette is placed in service and every six months thereafter. After the cassette has been loaded, it is placed on top of the cassette holder with the wire screen on top of it. The compression device, with acrylic sheets on top, if necessary, to assure an exposure time of at least 0.5 seconds, is placed as close to the X-ray tube as possible. After the film is exposed and processed, it is viewed at a distance of at least three feet. Darker areas indicate poor contact. Sources of the poor contact such as dust particles, cassette damage, or foam deterioration in the cassette should be identified and corrected or the cassette replaced.

View boxes and viewing conditions: All view boxes should be cleaned weekly with window cleaner and soft towels so that optimal viewing conditions are maintained. Mammography view boxes have a luminance level of at least 3000 candela/m^2, while those used in general radiology have lower levels on the order of 1500 candela/m^2. General light in the room should be at a low level and the area around mammograms masked to exclude extraneous light.

Repeat analysis: When mammograms are repeated or rejected, the process is inefficient, expensive, and increases patient exposure to radiation. Every three months, data on 250 consecutive patients should be collected. The total number of films taken during this time should also be calculated. Sort all the rejected films into the following standard categories: repeated because of positioning, patient motion, light films, dark films, black films, artifacts, fog, incorrect identification or double exposure, mechanical, miscellaneous, or good and without apparent reason for repeat and rejected because of clear films, wire localization, or quality control. Determine the overall percentage of repeated and rejected films as well as the percentage of each of the eleven repeat categories. MQSA requires that the overall repeat rate should be 2% or less. If a 5% rate is acceptable to the facility, then change from the previous rate of more than 2% should be investigated and corrective action taken.

Visual checklists: The mammography equipment must be stable and operate properly to ensure patient safety and high quality images, as well as operator convenience. A monthly checklist should be developed to include lights, displays, mechanical locks and detents on the C-arm and cassette holder and in the control booth. Individual items work or do not work and, those that do not should be repaired or replaced

Analysis of fixer retention on film: Residual fixer (hypo) on processed film indicates that the washing process is inadequate. The resulting brown stain degrades image stability. Every three months, a drop of the hypo solution should be placed on the emulsion side of an unexposed film, allowed to stand for 2 minutes, blotted, and the film placed on a sheet of white paper. The stain should be compared to a hypo estimator strip supplied by the manufacturer. The residual fixer should be no more than 5 micrograms per square cm. An identified problem must be corrected within 30 days.

Developer, fixer temperature, replacement rate: Manufacturer's recommendations for developer and fixer temperature should be followed. Low developer temperature results in decreased image contrast. Temperature should be measured with a digital thermometer (mercury should never be used because even traces will sensitize film) and compared with the reading on the built-in thermometer. The American College of Radiology recommends that the developer temperature should be within ± 0.5° F of manufacturer's recommendation and the fixer within ± 5.0° F of developer temperature. A true difference of more than 0.5° F in the developer will require the attention of a service engineer. Replenishment rates vary according to the film and processor used and checking requires training by the manufacturer while the equipment and procedures are specified in the training manual. The proper replenishment rate insures appropriate solution tank operating levels and proper film speed and film contrast.

Phantom Images

According to the American College of Radiology, the use of standard phantom images ensures that the film's optical density, contrast, uniformity, and image quality are maintained at optimum levels. The procedure should be done at least weekly, after service to any of the equipment, when the film or screen type is changed, or when problems are suspected. Place the mammography phantom on the cassette holder, lower the compression paddle, expose and process the film. Measure background optical density at the geographic center of the phantom image. Determine density difference (DD) by measuring optical density inside the disc and directly adjacent to the disc but perpendicular to the anode-cathode axis. The DD is the difference between the two measurements. Plot the background optical density and the DD on the control chart. Score the fibers, specks, and masses and circle any artifacts or grid lines on the film. Investigate the source of the latter.

The FDA-approved mammography phantom is approximately equivalent to a 4.2 cm thick breast consisting of 50% glandular and 50% adipose tissue. The wax insert includes a standard pattern of five fibers varying in diameter from 0.40 mm to 1.56 mm, five groups of specks ranging in diameter from 0.16 mm to 0.54 mm, and five masses with diameter ranging from 0.25 mm to 2.00 mm. A 4 mm thick acrylic disc for contrast measurement is glued in place on the surface between and slightly below the two largest fibers.

The interpretation of phantom images is most reliable when it is done by the same individual using the same criteria. The same view box, the same viewing conditions (e.g. time of day), and the same magnification must also be consistent. The same phantom and acrylic disc should also be used and all units at the facility should produce similar film optical densities, DD, and images. Images should be saved for comparison.

Standard scoring requires that each object type be scored separately and the number of visible objects be counted from the largest downward. Each fiber receives one point if the full length is visible and the location and orientation are correct. A fiber receives 0.5 points if more than half, but not all, is visible. If a fiber-like artifact appears on the image, deduct that from the last "real" whole or half fiber recorded. Specks are visualized with a magnifying lens (2x or higher). A speck group receives one point if four or more of the six specks in the group are visible in the proper location. A speck group receives 0.5 points if 2 or 3 of the six specks in the group are visible in the proper location. If speck-like artifacts are visible in the wrong locations, deduct them one-for-one from the individual specks counted in the last whole or half speck group scored. A mass receives one point if it appears in the correct location, is generally circular in appearance, and at least ¾ of the perimeter is visible. A mass receives 0.5 points if visible but without a generally circular shape. If a mass-like artifact is seen, it is deducted from the score. At this time, the image is also carefully observed with a magnifying glass for other artifacts or grid lines.

American College of Radiology standards for accreditation of phantom images require that, at a minimum, the four largest fibers, three largest speck groups, and three largest masses should be visualized and the number of items in each group should not decrease by more than half the original image. The phantom image background density should be at least 1.40 and not vary more than ± 0.20 from the operating level. The density difference from the acrylic disc should be at least 0.40 and not vary more than ± 0.05 from the operating level. Changes in image quality may be due to any component of the system, so if phantom image test scores fall outside the action limits, then testing will be needed to determine if the source of the problem is the X-ray generator, filter, film, cassette, screen processor, or view box.

Mobile Mammography Units

Mobile mammography units must meet the same requirements as stationary units and must be tested each time they are moved to different locations. Ideally, a phantom image is produced and evaluated before clinical exams are done. If the phantom image cannot be processed before mammograms are performed, then the measured radiation output of data from post-exposure mAs display must be within ± 10% of the established operating level in order to proceed.

Infection Control

Universal standard precautions should be utilized to control the spread of infection within the facility. Barrier protection (gowns and gloves) should be used if there is potential for contact with any moist surface on a patient's body. Staff should wash hands between patient contacts, wipe clean with approved disinfectant any surfaces in contact with the patient, disinfect any spills or drops on the floor, and change all linens after each patient. Patients in isolation should be scheduled to ensure the least exposure to others. Staff should have annual testing for tuberculosis and not have patient contact if they have an active infection of any kind.

Medical Physicist and Quality Assurance

The medical physicist's primary role is to assess the continuing performance of screen-film mammography equipment. He conducts a number of tests and then conveys the written test results to the facility so that corrective action can be taken. Significant problems should be noted before the medical physicist leaves the facility so that corrective action can be completed before the 30 days allotted by the Mammography Quality Standards Act. The medical physicist can also review the quality control testing and documentation done by the radiation technologists and provide an independent check on these tests.

Annual Quality Control Tests

Unit assembly evaluation: The physicist verifies that the mechanical components of the unit are operating properly. The unit is stable and does not wobble or vibrate. Moving parts operate without friction and cushions, bumper, locks, and detents limit motion appropriately. Indicator lights work properly. Adequate radiation shielding during exposure protects the operator. There should be no electrical or physical hazards (e.g. sharp edges) to patient or operator. Technologist charts are current, accurate, and posted. If the system provides for automatic decompression after exposure or power failure, then it must be tested to confirm an override capability to allow maintenance of compression if necessary, a continuous display of that override status, and a manual emergency compression release that can be activated in the event of power or automatic release failure.

System resolution: A standard resolution pattern is fixed 4.5 cm above the breast support plate. The pattern's bars lie parallel to the anode-cathode axis for the first image and perpendicular to that axis with the highest line frequency of the bar pattern toward the chest wall for the second. Exposure is done with SID, AEC, kVp, mA, focal spot, and density control settings at the most common clinical settings. Magnification is used to determine the highest frequency pattern whose lines are distinctly visible throughout at least half the bar length. MQSA requires that the system provide a resolution of 13 line-pairs/mm when the bars are parallel to the axis and11 line-pairs/mm when perpendicular.

Collimation assessment: The collimator provides an absorption boundary so that the X-ray field aligns with the collimator light field but radiation does not extend beyond its edges. In order to test this, film is exposed with four coins to mark the edges of the collimator light field and another at the chest wall edge of the compression paddle. After the film is exposed, the deviation between the X-ray field and the edge of the light field is measured. The sum of the four edge deviations is expressed as a percentage of the unit source-to-image distance (SID). MQSA requires that the X-ray field should not extend beyond the four sides of the image detector by more than 2% of SID. The chest wall edge of the compression paddle should not extend beyond the chest wall edge of the image receptor by more than 1% of SID.

Uniformity of screen speed: The screen speed of all cassettes in use should be uniform. With a 4 cm-thick, cassette-sized phantom, under commonly used control settings, all cassettes are exposed. The first cassette becomes the control as it is reloaded with new film in the middle and again at the end of the sequence. The standard deviation of the measured optical density at the center of the phantom for the three controls should not exceed 0.05. The maximum and minimum optical densities for all cassettes of a single size or type are then determined. MQSA requires that the difference between these shall not exceed 0.30. If no identified cause for deviation outside that range is found, then the cassette should be discarded. Screen artifacts should also be evaluated during this test.

Automatic exposure control (AEC) performance: The mammography unit must be able to maintain consistent image optical density with breasts of different thickness and different imaging modes. The density control selector function alters that optical density. Using clinically appropriate target material, filter, kVp, and density control settings, expose phantoms that are 2, 4, 6, and 8 cm thick. Measure the optical image density at the center of each phantom. Using the 4 cm thick phantom, repeat exposure for all the clinically used settings of the AEC's density control selector and again measure the image optical density at the center of the phantom. MQSA requires that the AEC should be capable of maintaining film optical density within ±0.15 of the mean optical density for all exposures and it shall not be less than 1.20.

Image quality evaluation: The annual test for image quality is the same as the technologist's weekly test for phantom image quality. It is performed using a mammography phantom with a standard pattern of fibers, specks, and masses. MQSA requires that, at a minimum, the four largest fibers, three largest specks, and three largest masses should be visualized and the number of items in each group should not decrease by more than half the original image. The phantom image background density should be at least 1.40 and not vary more than ± 0.20 from the operating level. The density difference from the acrylic disc should be at least 0.40 and not vary more than ± 0.05 from the operating level.

Screen artifact evaluation: Screen artifacts can be tested for at the same time that uniformity of screen speed is tested. A 4 cm-thick, cassette-size phantom is used. The control films are taken first with a lead arrow marker along the long axis of the film and cassette and then with the marker along the short axis. The films are processed with the arrows going in the same direction. The American College of Radiology notes that any artifacts running parallel in the two films are due to the processor (e.g. defective roller) while artifacts perpendicular in the two films are due to problems in the X-ray equipment or cassette (e.g. grid, image receptor holder, compression paddle, collimator, filter, X-ray tube). Changing one component at a time can help determine the source of the artifact.

Beam quality assessment (half value layer [HVL] assessment): The half value layer (HVL) of the X-ray beam should minimize patient breast dose without loss of contrast. A series of 0.1mm thick sheets of 99.9% pure aluminum (type 1145 aluminum alloy) is placed between an ionization chamber 4.5 cm above the image receptor holder and the source of the X-ray beam. Sheets are added until the exposure reading is less than one half the original exposure reading with no sheets. After calculation, the measured HVL must be greater than or equal the kVp divided by 100 plus 0.03 in units of mm of aluminum.

Kilovolt peak (kVp) accuracy and reproducibility: With the appropriate test device, make four exposures using the most commonly used clinical kilovolt peak (kVp) and other exposures including the lowest clinically used kVp that can be measured by the kVp test device and the highest available clinical kVp. MQSA requires that, at the most commonly used clinical setting, the coefficient of variation of reproducibility (standard deviation divided by average value) shall be equal to or less than 0.02. If it is greater than 0.02 or if the average measured kVp differs by more than ± 5% from the nominal kVp setting, then a service engineer should check the unit.

Radiation output rate: An ionization chamber is positioned 4.5 cm above the breast support plate and centered 4 cm from the chest wall. Record measured exposure and exposure time for this and all other clinically used SID settings. The system shall be capable of producing a minimum output of 7.0 mGy air kerma per second (800 mR per second) when operating at 28 kVp in the standard mammography mode (Mo/Mo) at any SID where the system is designed to operate. The system shall also be capable of maintaining the required minimum output averaged over a 3.0 second period.

Breast entrance exposure, automatic exposure control reproducibility, and average glandular dose: An ionization chamber/electrometer is positioned adjacent to a phantom and at the same height on the image receptor holder assembly. The compression paddle is put in place and commonly used clinical settings of kVp, target material, and filtration are utilized. Four exposures are made and the mean values for exposure and exposure time are calculated. Breast entrance air kerma (mGy/s) is equal to the exposure rate (mR/s) times the conversion factor (0.00873 mGy/mR). MQSA requires that the coefficient of variation for both air kerma and mAs shall not exceed 0.05. Average glandular dose is calculated using appropriate tables and, during a single cranio-caudal view of an FDA-approved phantom simulating a standard breast, shall not exceed 3.0 mGy (0.3 rad) per exposure.

View box luminance and room illuminance: Viewing conditions are optimized when the luminance from the view box is maximized and the ambient light in the room is minimized. Under normal lighting conditions in the viewing room, a photometer detector is placed parallel to and facing the view box surface within a soft, black rubber shade in contact with the view box surface. The American College of Radiology recommends that the view box should produce a luminance of at least 3.000 candela per square meter. The photometric detector with cosine diffuser rather than lens is then placed parallel to and facing away from the view box, but in contact with it. The illumination level in the room should be less than 50 lux.

Mammography Quality Standards Act (MQSA)

The MQSA establishes performance standards that a mammography facility must meet in order to operate lawfully. These standards include periodic review of clinical images, an annual survey by a medical physicist, and federal quality standards. The latter standards cover personnel, equipment, radiation dose, quality assurance programs, record keeping and reporting. A facility applies for certification by the Food and Drug Administration or qualified states as certifiers (SAC). Iowa, Illinois, and South Carolina are approved to certify facilities within those states. Provisional certification is granted for 6 months until the facility is accredited by an appropriate body, either the private, non-profit American College of Radiology, or the states of Arkansas, Iowa, or Texas. Certification is good for 3 years.

Personnel: MQSA requires that all personnel have individual records that document their licensure or certification, training in specific techniques, continuing experience, and continuing education. There must be a roster that includes the names and particular assignments of those responsible for quality assurance.

Record keeping: MQSA requires that each patient have a unique identification number and that it be displayed on all films. Films should be kept for 5 years (10 if no other mammogram is available or longer if required by state law.) Within days, each patient should receive a summary of the findings written in language easily understood by someone with no knowledge of medical terminology. The referring physician should also receive the findings within 30 days. A summary should be sent as soon as possible (3 to 5 days) if suggestive of malignancy. Reports should use standard assessment categories: negative, benign, probably benign, suspicious abnormality, highly suggestive for malignancy, known biopsy proven malignancy, or incomplete and in need of additional image evaluation.

Consumer complaints: MQSA requires that there be written documentation of a system for recording, maintaining for at least 3 years, and resolving consumer complaints. There must be written instructions for patients explaining how they should proceed to complain to the accreditation body if the complaint cannot be resolved by the facility.

Medical audits: MQSA requires that a designated auditing physician review all positive mammograms and attempt to obtain biopsy results to correlate with the radiographic findings. The audit should be done for each interpreting physician and for the facility as a whole.

Anatomy, Physiology, and Pathology

Clock Face and Quadrant Terminology

Each breast may be viewed as the face of a clock with the nipple at the center and points of interest located at one of the 12 hourly positions. Alternatively, the breast may be divided into 4 quadrants: upper outer (UOQ), upper inner (UIQ), lower outer (LOQ), and lower inner (LIQ). The clock face system is used to identify points of interest for magnification or follow-up. The less specific quadrant system is used in staging a malignancy e.g. ductal carcinoma is considered multifocal if all lesions are in the same quadrant and multicentric if more than one quadrant is involved. Most cancers occur in the UOQ. It is important to remember that a point of interest at 10 o'clock would be in the UOQ of the right breast but in the UIQ of the left.

Internal Anatomy

The subcutaneous area or stroma supporting the breast tissue itself contains fat or adipose tissue, connective tissue, blood vessels, nerves, and lymphatics. The breast tissue parenchyma consists of thousands of milk-secreting alveoli. Ten to 100 alveoli make up a lobule and 20 to 40 lobules make up a lobe. Collecting ducts from the 10 to 20 lobes open into the subareolar lactiferous sinuses. Ducts from these sinuses open at the nipple. The breast tissue is separated from the pectoralis muscle by the retromammary space, a layer of fatty tissue.

External Anatomy

The adult female breast is suspended between the 2nd and 4th ribs in the vertical plane and the outer edge of the sternum and the mid-axillary line in the horizontal plane. Breast tissue extends upward from the submammary or inframammary fold into the axilla as the axillary tail of Spence, the densest part of the breast. The skin contains hair follicles, sebaceous (oil producing) glands, and sweat glands. The nipple is usually in the 4th intercostal space in a non-pendulous breast. The nipple has sensory nerve endings and sebaceous and sweat glands, but no hair follicles. The nipple is surrounded by the circular pigmented areola which is usually 15-60 mm in diameter. The areola contains Morgagni tubercles.

Blood Flow

Approximately 60% of the blood supply to the breast comes from the anterior perforating branches on the internal mammary artery. These supply the medial and central portions of the breast. Thirty percent, the supply to the upper outer quadrant, comes from the lateral thoracic artery. The rest is made up of small amounts supplied by the pectoral branch of the thoracoacromial artery, branches of the 3rd, 4th, and 5th intercostal arteries, subcapsular, and thoracodorsal arteries. Veins are larger and more superficial than arteries and drain into the axillary and internal mammary veins.

Fascial Tissue

Fascia is a sheet of fibrous tissue beneath the skin and surrounding muscles. The superficial pectoral fascia envelops the breast, and is continuous with the superficial abdominal fascia of Camper. The undersurface of the breast lies on the deep pectoral fascia that covers the pectoralis major and anterior serratus muscles. Fibrous bands connect these two fascial layers. These Cooper suspensory ligaments provide support to the breast.

Musculature

There is no muscle tissue in the breast. The breast lies on the pectoralis major muscle. This superficial chest muscle has its origin on the medial half of the clavicle, the sternum, and cartilages of the 1st through 6th ribs and its insertion on the crest of the greater tubercle of the humerus. The pectoralis minor is a deeper muscle, as is the serratus anterior.

Lymphatic Drainage

97% of lymphatic drainage is to the axillary nodes and 3% to the internal mammary nodes. There are many arbitrary ways of dividing the axillary nodes – one differentiates those nodes lateral to the lateral border of the pectoralis minor muscle from those behind that muscle and those medial to its medial border. Lymph nodes are kidney shaped and less than 2 cm in size.

Terminal Ductal Lobular Unit (TDLU)

The terminal ductal lobular unit (TDLU) consists of a breast lobule and its associated ducts and is the primary functioning unit of the breast. The lobule consists of approximately 11 alveoli (also called acini or ductules) surrounded by connective tissue. That portion of the collecting duct within the lobule is called the intralobular duct and the portion outside the lobule emptying into the duct to the lobe is the extralobular duct. Epithelial cells line the ductal system.

The epithelium, an avascular cellular lining of the TDLU, consists of the outermost myoepithelial cells, and the inner luminal epithelial cells supported by a basement membrane. During lactation, the luminal cells secrete milk and the myoepithelial cells contract to aid in ejection of the milk. The basement membrane is a matrix of collagen and glycoproteins that supports the epithelium and acts as a selective filter. Most breast malignancies arise from the TDLU epithelium and changes in myoepithelial cell function appear to play a major role in the development of cancer.

Morgagni Tubercles and Montgomery Glands

Morgagni tubercles are located near the outer edge of the areola and are small, rounded projections formed by the openings of the ducts of the Montgomery glands. The Montgomery glands, also known as the areolar glands, enlarge during pregnancy and, during lactation, secrete a substance presumed to protect the areola during suckling.

Viewing Mammograms

Mass: A mass is a space-occupying lesion visible on two different projections. Masses are characterized by shape, margin, and density. There are many exceptions, but round or oval shapes are more likely to be benign than are irregular or lobular ones. Similarly, circumscribed, well-defined margins are more likely to be benign than are indistinct or microlobulated ones. A star-like pattern of radiating lines has the highest risk of malignancy. A halo effect is typical of benign lesions, but it is not always present. Density may vary from the non-absorption characteristic of fat, through moderate tissue absorption, to the high absorption characteristic of calcification.

Oil cysts: When fat tissue in the breast dies (usually as a result of trauma to the breast), the necrotic tissue changes to oil, a process known as aseptic saponification. The body then forms a capsule around it. On a mammogram, an oil cyst would appear as a high density mass with liquid in a central cavity and egg shell-like calcification in the capsule. The benign cyst may be fixed to surrounding tissue.

Cysts: A cyst is defined as a sac that has a membranous lining or capsule and that contains a fluid or semisolid material. In the breast, a cyst may develop if an extralobular terminal duct is blocked and fluid accumulated behind that blockage. This would appear as a translucent mass on a mammogram. By definition, oil cysts and galactoceles are also cysts.

Galactoceles: A galactocele is a small milk-filled cyst due to an obstructed milk duct. It occurs during lactation or after breast-feeding has ended. On mammography it may appear as a round or oval lesion with a well-circumscribed wall or as an indeterminate mass. There may be a fat-fluid level. A galactocele is benign.

Lipomas: Lipomas are benign fatty tumors that can occur in the breast and may or may not be encapsulated by scar tissue or a thin layer of connective tissue. Like all fat deposits, they appear dark on mammography.

Fibroadenomas: A fibroadenoma is a benign mass that includes both glandular and connective tissue. It is often pseudo-encapsulated and sharply delineated from the surrounding breast tissue. Fibroadenomas range in size from very small to several inches across and are most common in women between 20 and 40.

Papillomas: A papilloma is a benign tumor of the lactiferous ducts. It may cause a bloody nipple discharge. Hyperplastic epithelium covers tree-like fronds of fibrovascular stroma that are attached to the wall of the duct by a stalk. Papillomas are not visualized on mammography unless contrast material is introduced via ductography.

Hamartomas: A hamartoma is a mass containing a variable amount of glandular tissue, fibrous connective tissue, and fat. It is most commonly found in post-menopausal women. It is visualized as a well-circumscribed lesion containing both fat and tissue densities, surrounded by a capsule best seen in a projection where there is fat on both sides of it. A poorly visualized or atypical presentation usually requires excision of the mass.

Hematomas: A hematoma is a blood clot that occurs after trauma or surgery on the breast. It presents as an ill-defined mass that typically increases in size immediately after the trauma and then resolves and grows smaller. A mass of mixed density would appear on mammography.

Ductal ectasias: Ductal ectasia is a benign dilation of the subareolar ducts and is most common in women over 50. It may be a source of nipple discharge or be accompanied by a variety of changes including inflammation. Ductal ectasia is not visualized on mammography unless contrast material is introduced via ductography. It appears as dilation of the lumen of the duct without the filling defect characteristic of a papilloma.

Radial scars: A radial scar contains a central fibroelastic core. The core contains scattered bits of glandular tissue. Radiating from the core are ducts and lobules that may show changes ranging from cysts to hyperplasia. A radial scar with multiple, needle-like projections may be confused with malignancy. These scars may be associated with an increased risk of malignancy and should be monitored closely for changes.

Breast abscesses: A breast abscess or pocket of pus may be part of an acute inflammatory process. It is characterized by pain, tenderness, and redness along with fever and chills. An abscess should respond to a course of appropriate antibiotic or may require lancing and drainage. On mammography, the poorly defined mass should shrink with treatment.

Lymph nodes: Intramammary lymph nodes are seen on 5-8% of routine mammograms. Most appear round or oval and have sharply outlined margins. They are most commonly found in the Upper Outer Quadrant and axillary tail of the breast. They have a radiolucent center at the hilum, the fatty center where lymphatics and vessels enter and leave the node.

Benign calcifications: Benign calcifications tend to be sharply outlined and round or oval in shape with smooth contours and high uniform density. Some shapes are characteristic, such as pear-shaped milk of calcium, ring-shaped sebaceous gland calcification, or eggshell-like oil cyst calcification. Calcification that is bilateral and evenly scattered is likely to be benign as are large, unusually shaped calcification as seen is a resolved hematoma.

Invasive ductal carcinomas: Invasive ductal carcinoma or infiltrating ductal carcinoma is the most common form on invasive breast carcinoma and accounts for 70% of these cases. Invasive ductal carcinoma originates within the ducts in the breast but breaks through the wall and infiltrates the surrounding tissue. It may also metastasize via blood and lymph to other sites in the body, particularly the regional lymph nodes. On mammography, the borders appear to be irregular and microcalcifications are almost always present.

Ductal carcinoma in situ: Ductal carcinoma in situ (DCIS) describes a cancer that has not spread beyond the duct by invading the surrounding tissue. DCIS is the most common type of invasive breast cancer and accounts for 25% of all breast cancer diagnoses. About one fourth of the breast cancer detected by mammography is DCIS because almost 90% of DCIS lesions contain microcalcifications. Microcalcifications are tiny specks of calcium that follow cell death and are clustered at the site of DCIS.

Inflammatory breast carcinomas: Inflammatory breast carcinoma is an uncommon but rapidly progressive tumor. It is characterized by firm, painful swelling and reddish-purple discoloration of the breast and swollen lymph nodes. Ductal carcinoma cells embolize in the lymphatic channels and capillaries become engorged. There is no characteristic picture on mammography.

Invasive lobular carcinomas: Invasive lobular carcinoma accounts for 5-10% of invasive breast tumors. Often it occurs in several sites in the same breast (multicentricity) and 30% of the time in the contralateral breast as well. Margins are poorly defined and this lesion often presents with skin thickening without specific findings on mammography. There may be only a dense area, and microcalcifications are found in only 5% of cases.

Sarcomas: Mammary angiosarcomas or endovascular tumors are rare and account for less than 1% of breast tumors. They are generally found in women age 20 to 40 but may also occur in older women in tissue that has been irradiated for breast cancer or in lymphedematous areas after mastectomy. These tumors present as poorly defined masses and show no specific findings on mammography. They may include coarse calcifications.

Paget's disease: In Paget's disease of the nipple, malignant cells from the duct migrate to the skin of the nipple and areola which then show eczematous changes. The skin appears crusted, scaly and red and there may be associated oozing or bleeding from the nipple. Mammographic findings depend on the underlying pathology, either ductal carcinoma in situ or invasive ductal carcinoma.

Malignant calcifications: Calcifications that are malignant may present in linear, fragmented, or occasionally branching patterns in ductal carcinoma in situ. There may be clusters of granules of various forms, size, and density or multiple clusters of powdery calcifications.

Lymphoma: Primary breast lymphoma within a mammary lymph node is extremely rare. On a mammogram it would appear as a well-circumscribed nodular density.

Stellate masses: Stellate ("star-like") or speculated ("needle-like") masses are commonly associated with malignancy and are often accompanied by malignant calcification. On mammography, they present as a distinct central mass with sharp lines of variable length radiating in all directions. If a spike reaches the skin, it may cause local thickening or dimpling.

Lactating Women

During lactation, the increased blood supply and milk production result in increased glandularity that makes interpretation difficult. Radiation exposure is also increased. A mammogram should not be scheduled during lactation unless the woman is symptomatic or has a history of breast cancer and is at high risk.

Mammographic Technique and Image Evaluation

The radiologist must evaluate clinical images every day as part of the quality control program required for facility accreditation. Each mammogram should be assessed for technical deficiencies such as breast positioning, compression, image quality, and artifacts. The technologist should receive feedback about defective images and the causes of image deficiencies should be identified and addressed as quickly as possible.

Kilovolt Peak (kVp)

The kilovolt peak (kVp) determines the maximum energy of X-rays emitted by the tube. For mammography, an operating voltage below 35 kVp provides sufficient penetration without excessive exposure time. The Mo/Mo peak is sufficient for thin breasts, Mo/Rh for thicker and denser breasts, and Rh/Rh for the thickest, densest breasts. Any increase in kVp increases Compton scatter but also decreases exposure time and dose.

Density Setting

Optical density is determined by a combination of amperage and exposure. To achieve a density of 1.5 to 2.0 with constant amperage, the exposure will vary depending on the tissue being imaged. The automatic exposure control (AEC) is placed under the densest part of the breast in order to provide optimal penetration and a sharp image. The AEC provides correction for reciprocity failure due to light exposure from the intensifying screens at very long and very short exposure settings.

Milliampere-Seconds (mAs)

Milliampere-seconds (mAs) are the product of the electron current (mA) within the tube and the exposure time in seconds. For fixed kVp, the total X-ray output is linearly proportional to mAs. Tube current is usually 100 mA (± 25 mA) for a large focal spot and 25 mA (± 10 mA) for a small focal spot. A reasonable exposure time ranges from 0.5 to 2.0 seconds to achieve an optical density of 1.5 – 2.0.

Compression

Compression should be applied to the maximum degree to which the patient's breast can be compressed and which is tolerable to the patient without being painful. Too little compression results in a poor image despite a higher dose of radiation. Too much compression may damage breast tissue and discourage the patient from having further mammograms. The compressed breast should be taut so that gentle pressure does not cause an indentation in the skin.

Compression reduces the thickness of the breast so that X-rays penetrate uniformly. Compression separates structures within the breast and facilitates the distinction of areas of interest. Proper compression reduces the dose of X-ray needed for adequate exposure and improves contrast by decreasing scattered radiation. Immobilization of the breast by the compression device also lessens the chance of motion blurring.

Patients may be able to tolerate more compression if they are prepared for it and it is applied slowly. If the patient understands the need for compression and how long it will be applied, then she may tolerate more. Patients with very sensitive breasts make take a mild analgesic such as ibuprofen prior to mammography. If a woman's breasts are particularly sensitive during menstruation, then the mammogram should be scheduled at some other time in the menstrual cycle.

MAGNIFICATION MAMMOGRAPHY

With magnification of the image 1.5 – 2 times, small areas such as microcalcifications, surgical sites, and excised specimens can be better visualized. The margins of suspicious lesions and the number, form, and distribution of microcalcifications may be seen more clearly. A small focal spot must be used with magnification in order to maintain the sharpness of the image. A small compression paddle is also used. The large air gap reduces scatter.

In magnification mammography, the breast is closer to the X-ray source and therefore receives a higher dose of radiation. Without a small focal spot, there is geometric blurring. The longer exposure time for magnification provides the potential for patient motion and subsequent blurring. In a magnified view the location, density, and size of a lesion cannot be assessed relative to the whole breast.

A grid is unnecessary in magnification mammography because the air gap as a result of larger object-image-distance already reduces the amount of scattered radiation reaching the film. If a grid were to be used, it would increase exposure time thereby increasing both the potential for motion artifact and the radiation dose.

IMAGE QUALITY

Mediolateral oblique (MLO) positioning: The MLO view should visualize as much breast tissue as possible. To assure this, the pectoralis muscle should be visualized down to the posterior nipple line. If the retroglandular fat is visible, then all the fibroglandular tissue is probably included. An open inframammary fold assures that the lower posterior breast tissue is adequately visualized. A large 24 x 30 cm receptor will provide adequate visualization of axillary tissue and inferior breast tissue in a large breast and an 18 x 24 cm receptor will assure adequate compression in a small breast. MQSA requires that at least both of these size plates must be available.

Compression: Insufficient compression will result in one breast structure superimposed on another, variable exposure and penetration, and blurring secondary to motion. Inadequate compression in the MLO view may result in sagging or "camel's nose" appearance. If extraneous axillary or abdominal tissue is compressed in the MLO view, then the breast itself will not be fully compressed. Other causes of poor compression may be a faulty compression device or inadequate force applied by the technologist.

Craniocaudal (CC) positioning: The CC view should visualize as much posteromedial breast tissue as possible because this is the area most often missed in the MLO view. The ACR Quality Control Manual states that if the pectoralis muscle is visible or if "the posterior nipple line is within 1 cm of its length in the MLO view," then adequate posterior tissue has been included. All the fibroglandular tissue in the medial aspect of the breast should be included even if all the lateral tissue is not. The position of the nipple in views of both breasts should be consistent.

Contrast: The American College of Radiology defines "contrast" as the difference in optical density between adjacent areas of film. This is usually a problem in thicker breasts because of greater radiation scatter and absorption of low kVp radiation. The ACR Quality Control Manual notes that poor compression, overexposure or underexposure, use of low-contrast film, processing error, inappropriate target material and/or filtration, failure to use a grid, and excessive kVp can all result in poor contrast.

Exposure: Underexposure results in decreased radiographic contrast whenever optical densities within breast tissue are below 1.0. This limits the ability to visualize fine details such as microcalcifications. Overexposure is seen when there is too much blackening of skin or fatty areas. While overexposed views may be "recovered" with higher illumination, underexposure is not recoverable. Underexposure may result from poor function or placement of the automatic exposure control, inadequate compression, or processing error.

Noise: Noise or "mottle" is seen as a lack of homogeneity in the background density. As a result, it is difficult to visualize tiny structures such as calcifications. This may be due to quantum mottle which the American College of Radiology defines as "the statistical fluctuation in the number of X-ray photons absorbed at individual locations on the intensifying screen." The fewer the photons making up the image, the greater the probability that quantum mottle will occur. Underexposure, extended processing, and faster image receptors are all associated with fewer photons. Fluctuations in film grain and processing may also produce noise.

Sharpness: "Unsharpness" means that adjacent structures that should be clearly differentiated are blurry instead. Motion blur is usually unidirectional and due to inadequate compression. Localized unsharpness may be due to poor screen-film contact as a result of cassette damage or dirt or air between the screen and the film. Geometric unsharpness is mild and generalized and the result of an increase in focal spot size or object-to-image receptor distance or a decrease in source-to-image receptor distance. Parallax unsharpness is blurring as a result of using double emulsion film where the image on each side of the film is separated by the width of the film.

Collimation: MQSA requires that the collimation field should extend slightly beyond the edge of the film on the chest wall side, but by not more than 2% of the source-to-image distance The X-ray beam is collimated as close to the edges of the film as possible and not to the surface of the breast. The latter would result in the exclusion of some breast tissue as well as clear areas on the film.

Artifacts: The American College of Radiology defines an artifact as "any density variation on an image that does not reflect true attenuation differences in the subject." Dust and dirt reflect a problem in darkroom cleanliness, scratches and fingerprints a problem in film handling, and fog an indication of light leaks. Grid lines are due to a faulty grid or processor. Roller marks from a processor tend to be wider, fewer in number, and spaced farther apart than grid lines.

Labels

MQSA strongly **recommends** a flash card patient identification system, which then becomes a permanent part of the image and is reproduced on copy films. The flash label should have a designated space near the edge of the film.

MQSA recommends separate date stickers that can be read by overhead light and may be color-coded by year for quick reference. It is also recommended that technical factors appear on the film. If target/filter, kVp, mAs, exposure time, compression force, compressed breast thickness, and degree of obliquity are noted, then they can be reproduced in subsequent films.

MQSA **requires** that each image has a label that contains the facility name, facility location, patient name, patient identification number, and date of examination. A marker indicating right or left breast and the view in standard abbreviation should be placed near that aspect of the breast tissue nearest the axilla. The technologist must be identified as well as the screen (usually as an Arabic numeral) and mammography unit (usually as a Roman numeral) if there is more than one unit at the facility.

Positioning and Interventional Procedures

The mediolateral oblique (MLO) and craniocaudal (CC) views are generally the only views taken for a screening examination. They take advantage of the mobility of the breast to maximize the amount of tissue that can be seen. The glandular and fatty tissue on the lateral and inferior parts of the breast can be compressed while the medial and superior aspects are fixed to the chest wall. In the standard views, the compression plate takes advantage of the mobile margins. The standard nomenclature for views places the location of the source before the location of the receptor.

Mediolateral Oblique (MLO) View

For the MLO view, the cassette holder is parallel to the edge of the pectoral muscle with the corner of the image receptor in the posterior part of the axilla. Patients of average height and weight require an angle of 40° - 50° from the horizontal; tall, thin patients require a steeper angle of 50° - 60°; short, heavy patients require a narrower angle between 30° and 40°. The X-ray beam is directed from the superomedial to the inferolateral aspect of the breast. This view maximizes the amount of breast tissue seen with the shortest object-to-image distance and the best resolution in the area most susceptible to malignancy.

When the MLO view is optimal, the pectoral muscle is wider at the top of the image and presents a convex anterior border extending to or below an imaginary line drawn from the nipple back to the chest wall. Retromammary fat is visible behind the breast tissue and the breast tissue itself is well separated. The inframammary fold is open and there is no evidence of motion blur.

After the cassette holder is in place, the technologist holds the breast out and up, away from the chest wall, as the compression paddle is lowered. The hand moves anteriorly as the paddle maintains the breast in this position. This provides adequate tissue separation and prevents downward sagging of the breast, the so-called "camel's nose" appearance. Finally, the abdominal tissue is pulled down to open the inframammary fold.

90° Lateral View

The 90° lateral views are used along with the standard MLO views to localize a lesion in the breast or to demonstrate gravity-dependent calcifications. The ACR *Quality Control Manual* indicates that if the lesion is higher on the lateral view than it is on the MLO view, then it is in the medial aspect of the breast. If the lesion is lower on the lateral view than it is on the MLO view, then it is in the lateral aspect of the breast. If the lesion does not move, then it is in the central aspect of the breast. The medial-to-lateral (ML) or lateral-to-medial (LM) view is then used so that the lesion is closest to the cassette holder for maximum sharpness.

Craniocaudal (CC) View

For the CC view, the cassette holder is placed in the inframammary fold after the breast is raised as high as mobility allows. The breast is pulled away from the chest wall with one of the technologist's hands on top of the breast and the other under it. The breast is positioned on the cassette holder with the nipple in the center.

The patient turns so that the cassette holder is flush against the sternum, the contralateral breast is draped over the corner of the cassette, and the patient moves her head forward. The technologist then lifts the posterior lateral aspect of the breast and pulls the breast forward and smoothes lateral tissue to eliminate folds as the compression paddle is lowered. The CC view maximizes visualization of medial tissue that may not be seen in the MLO view.

Spot Compression

Spot compression may be helpful in clarifying questionable findings, particularly in dense tissue. Spot compression allows for greater reduction in breast tissue mass and a better separation of that tissue. With collimation to the spot, there is greater contrast within the area of concern. An appropriately sized spot compression device can be placed over the area of a possible lesion by using the triangulation technique.

Mediolateral (ML) and Lateromedial (LM) 90° Lateral Views

For the mediolateral (ML) view, the cassette holder is anchored in the axilla and the breast tissue and pectoral muscle are pulled anteriorly and medially. With the compression paddle against the sternum, the patient is rotated until the breast is centered on the cassette holder and the breast is then pulled forward while compression is applied. The inframammary fold is then pulled open. For the lateromedial (LM) view, the cassette holder is anchored at the sternum and the breast tissue is pulled anteriorly and medially. The compression paddle is brought past the latissimus dorsi muscle and the patient's arm rested upon it. The breast is pulled forward while compression is applied. The inframammary fold is then pulled open.

Magnification (M) Views

Magnification may be combined with spot compression to get a more precise view of a suspected lesion. One can then assess the edges and character of a mass or clarify the quantity, pattern, and shape of calcifications. The X-ray tube must have a small focal spot and the greater the magnification sought, the smaller the focal spot necessary to provide it. A magnification platform must be used between the breast and the cassette. The resulting air gap prevents scattered radiation from reaching the film so a grid is unnecessary.

Triangulation Technique

The triangulation technique can be utilized on either MLO or CC views. As described in the ACR *Quality Control* Manual, a line is first drawn directly posterior from the nipple. Then, the distance from that line to the lesion in either the superior-inferior or medial-lateral direction is measured as is the distance from the lesion to the skin surface. These three measurements are then marked on the breast and the spot compression device can then be centered on the suspected lesion.

Cleavage (CV) View

According to the ACR *Quality Control* Manual, the cleavage (CV) view is utilized to visualize deep lesions in the posterior-medial aspect of the breast. The patient turns her head away from the side of interest. The technologist elevates the inframammary folds and places both breasts on the cassette holder. The medial tissue of both breasts must then be pulled forward. If the photocell is under the breast of interest, automatic exposure may be used. If it is between the breasts, then manual exposure is required.

Exaggerated Craniocaudal (XCCL) View

According the ACR *Quality Control Manual,* an exaggerated craniocaudal view attempts to identify deep lesions in the outer aspect of the breast. The patient is positioned as for the CC view, but, after the inframammary fold is elevated, the patient is rotated so that the outer aspect of the breast, including most of the axillary tail, is on the cassette holder. The patient should hold both her shoulders at the same level so that the breast is not distorted.

Tangential (TAN) View

A tangential (TAN) view is used to visualize palpable lumps that are otherwise hidden by dense tissue on a standard view. A lead marker over the lump facilitates the placement of the X-ray beam tangential to that marker. Tangential views can also verify the location of calcifications within the skin. Again, a lead marker is placed over the calcifications and the beam is tangential to the marker.

Axillary Tail (AT) View

The axillary tail (AT) view visualized all the tissue in the axillary tail. The cassette holder is placed parallel to the axillary tail and the patient's arm is draped behind it. The technologist pulls the axillary tail away from the chest wall and holds it in place while compression is applied.

Caudocranial (FB) View

According to the ACR *Quality Control Manual*, the caudocranial (FB for "from below") view is used to improve visualization of points of interest in the uppermost aspect of the breast. These would then be closest to the film. The FB view maximizes the amount of tissue visible in a man or in a woman with kyphosis. The male breast may also need to be shaved as the compression device may slide off a hairy surface. The FB view also provides easier access for needle localization of an area of interest in the inferior part of the breast.

Roll View

A roll view is used to separate tissues that overlap on a standard view. The patient is positioned using the same view that showed a possible abnormality and the technologist then rolls the breast with her hands moving in opposite directions. The roll is then maintained by compression. The film should be marked with the original projection and the roll view as a suffix: rolled lateral (RL), rolled medial (RM), rolled superior (RS), rolled inferior (RI). The direction is the direction in which the upper surface is rolled.

Superolateral to Inferomedial Oblique (SIO) View

The SIO view with the beam directed from upper-outer to lower-inner puts the lower medial aspects of the breast closer to the film for better visualization. This view is not commonly used.

Lateromedial Oblique (LMO) View

According to the ACR *Quality Control Manual* the LMO view is the exact reverse of the MLO view with the beam directed from the lower-outer to upper-inner aspects of the breast. Medial breast tissue is closer to the film and is therefore better visualized. This view more comfortably positions the breast and visualizes more tissue in patients with chest deformities, recent open heart surgery, or a pacemaker.

Implant Displaced (IO) Views

Standard CC and MLO implant-included views of the breast require that the exposure be set manually. Compression is limited by the physical characteristics of the implant. In such cases, the implant is displaced backward and upward against the chest wall and the breast tissue is gently pulled forward onto the cassette holder and held in place by the compression paddle. That makes a total of 8 views rather than 4 for bilateral implants. If the implant is in front of the pectoral muscle rather than beneath it, capsular contraction may make displacement difficult. In that case, a 90° degree lateral view with implant included should be taken along with the CC and MLO implant-included views.

Breast Surgery Considerations

Mammograms after *lumpectomy* are usually taken as standard views with markers identifying the surgical site. Magnification may be required. Mammography after *mastectomy* is not universally recommended. If it is, standard views of the skin over the mastectomy site, a spot view of any area of concern, and an axillary tail view may be done.

After *breast reduction by tissue excision*, there may be benign calcifications within the skin at the incision site in the periareolar region. These can be monitored by mammography. *Breast reduction by liposuction* rather than tissue excision results in fewer parenchymal changes. Breast reduction does not interfere with mammography which may be even easier with a smaller breast.

Irradiated Breast

Mammograms are usually done 6 to 12 months after the completion of radiation treatment and the edema has subsided. The persistence of a mass 6 months after therapy suggests that the treatment has failed. In patients for whom physical examination is inadequate to assess tumor response, serial mammograms may be helpful.

Chest Wall Deformities or Kyphosis

The sternum is depressed in both kyphosis and pectus excavatum. A caudocranial (FB) view would include the most breast tissue. If the breasts can be imaged from above, two CC views are taken to see the lateral parts of each breast and a CV view is taken to visualize the medial aspects. The LMO rather than the MLO view is utilized because, in the former, the plate is pressed against the sternum.

Protruding Abdomen

A protruding abdomen may cover the inframammary fold and interfere with compression of the anterior part of the breast. The patient must lean forward over the cassette holder and the angle of the tube may have to be reduced in order to adequately image the entire breast.

Fine Needle Aspiration and Core Biopsy

Fine needle aspiration removes a few cells for examination through a 23 gauge needle. A core biopsy removes a larger sample with a spring-loaded 11-14 gauge needle. In both procedures mammography can be utilized to guide the needle to the area of concern. Localization may be facilitated by the use of computer generated coordinates of the suspected lesion.

Pacemaker or Infusaport Considerations

Pacemakers are usually placed in the pectoral region and may obscure part of a mammogram. They should be treated like implants and gently displaced if possible, without damaging the leads. An LMO projection would be most comfortable and less potentially damaging than compression from the medial side.

An infusaport, or permanent central venous catheter, would not interfere with a mammogram but care should be used around it when positioning the patient. Again, the LMO projection would be more comfortable and less potentially damaging than compression from the medial side.

Preoperative Needle Localization

When a lesion cannot be palpated, then a needle or wire may be placed in the lesion during mammography in order to assist the surgeon in locating and removing it. This procedure allows the surgeon to excise as small an area as possible but ensures that the specimen with wire intact is from the site of concern. The insertion should be done from the direction where the skin to lesion distance is the shortest to aid in accuracy.

Pneumocystography

After a breast cyst has been aspirated, air can be injected in order to evaluate the inner wall of the cyst. The needle is guided by mammography. The air is generally resorbed within a week.

Ductography

If there is an abnormal nipple discharge, then that milk duct can be cannulated and 1-5 cc of contrast material introduced. Mammographic views are taken in the CC and ML projections. The ductogram can help determine the number and location of lesions, but only a cytological examination can determine malignancy.

Breast Specimen Imaging

The specimen is that part of the breast removed during biopsy or surgery. When compared to the original mammogram, a mammogram of the specimen confirms that the area of concern has been removed and the margins are clean. Compression of the specimen provides uniform thickness and improves resolution. Magnification may aid in visualizing microcalcifications. The specimen should be viewed immediately upon receipt in case the surgeon needs to remove additional tissue and the patient is still under anesthesia.

Mammography Practice Test

1. A woman should be counseled to perform monthly breast self-exams beginning at age

a. 18
b. 20
c. 40
d. 50

2. Breast sonography is not appropriate for

a. Pregnant women
b. Women with dense breasts
c. Women with implants
d. Routine screening

3. Which of the following is NOT true of breast ductography?

a. A small needle removes material from a mass, which is smeared onto a slide for interpretation.
b. It is contraindicated in women who are allergic to contrast dye.
c. Mammography is performed to observe ductal obstructions or masses.
d. Contrast material is injected into the nipple ducts.

4. MRI with contrast is most useful in showing

a. Solid breast tumors
b. Tumors with increased blood flow
c. Fluid-filled masses
d. Microcalcifications

5. Early menopause and osteoporosis are side effects of

a. Tamoxifen
b. Chemotherapy
c. Radiation therapy
d. Mastectomy

6. The large focal spot is usually ___ millimeters in size.

a. 3.0
b. 1.0
c. 0.3
d. 0.1

7. The film cassette should be allowed to rest for ___ minutes before being exposed.

a. 5
b. 15
c. 30
d. 60

8. Compression force must be maintained between ___ and ___ lbs of force.

a. 10 and 20
b. 15 and 35
c. 25 and 45
d. 35 and 50

9. Women with thick or dense breasts need a ______ dose of radiation, requiring the technologist to _______ the kVp.

a. Lower ... lower
b. Lower ... raise
c. Higher ... lower
d. Higher ... raise

10. What controls the length of radiation exposure after the breast tissue has been sufficiently exposed to the radiation?

a. The anode
b. The AEC
c. The x-ray filter
d. The cathode

11. Which of the following is the distance from the source of the radiation to the image receptor?

a. Object–image-receptor distance
b. Source–object distance
c. Source–image distance
d. Focal-spot–image distance

12. What is the purpose of the grid?

a. To convert x rays to light photons
b. To improve contrast by decreasing radiation scatter
c. To show the location of the focal spot
d. For quality control purposes

13. The darkroom must be cleaned each day because

a. The presence of any dirt or dust may produce artifacts on the film
b. Of the risk of infection transmission
c. It can damage the development equipment
d. Of the potential for a reaction of the dirt with the developing chemicals

14. When is it NOT necessary to process phantom images as a part of quality control measures?

a. Weekly
b. After the equipment is serviced
c. After changing the type of film used
d. Monthly

15. Which of the following is NOT a characteristic of the FDA-approved phantom used for mammography?

a. 4.2 cm breast thickness
b. 25% glandular and 75% adipose tissue
c. The presence of five masses measuring between 0.25 and 2 mm
d. The presence of five fibers with a diameter between 0.4 and 1.56 mm

16. Which personal protective equipment should be used when performing mammography in an outpatient clinic?

a. Gloves, gown, and mask
b. Gloves and mask
c. Gloves, gown, and goggles
d. Gloves

17. How soon should the referring physician receive a copy of the findings if a malignancy is suspected?

a. 60 days
b. 30 days
c. 1 week
d. 3 to 5 days

18. Most breast cancers occur in which quadrant of the breast?

a. Upper outer
b. Upper inner
c. Lower outer
d. Lower inner

19. What type of tissue occupies the retromammary space?

a. Fatty tissue
b. Connective tissue
c. Lymphatics
d. Muscle

20. The breast is supported by tissue between which two ribs?

a. First and third
b. First and second
c. Second and fourth
d. Second and third

21. A majority of blood flow to the breast comes from the

a. Thoracoacromial artery
b. Thoracodorsal artery
c. Lateral thoracic artery
d. Internal mammary artery

22. Which muscle makes up the breast?

a. There is no muscle tissue in the breast
b. Pectoralis major muscle
c. Mammary muscle
d. Pectoralis minor

23. Which cells contract to aid in milk ejection?

a. Luminal cells
b. Epithelial cells
c. Myoepithelial cells
d. Extralobular ductal cells

24. Which structure secretes a protective substance that is used as a barrier to bacteria during nursing?

a. Montgomery glands
b. Morgagni tubercles
c. Myoepithelial cells
d. The alveoli

25. A cyst filled with milk is also called what?

a. A lipoma
b. An oil cyst
c. A papilloma
d. A galactocele

26. Which of the following is characteristic of a benign calcification on mammography?

a. Vague outline
b. Sharp edges
c. Irregular density
d. Sharp outline

27. Crusty, scaly skin on the areola with minor bleeding from the nipple indicates

a. Mammary endovascular tumor
b. Paget's disease
c. Ductal carcinoma *in situ*
d. Stellate mass

28. Exposure time should range between:

a. 0.5 and 2.0 sec
b. 1.0 and 3.0 sec
c. 1.5 and 2.5 sec
d. 2.0 and 4.0 sec

29. How can you tell if sufficient compression has been applied to the breast?

a. Skin color blanches.
b. The tissue is still soft and supple.
c. The skin is taut and does not dent when a finger is pressed into it.
d. The patient begins to complain of discomfort.

30. Compression of the breast

a. Keeps the breast at the proper physiological position during the exam
b. Allows the x ray to penetrate the tissue evenly
c. Keep the x-ray source and the image close enough together
d. Forces masses to become more visible on the outside of the breast

31. During magnification mammography, the image is magnified by how many times?

a. 2
b. 5
c. 10
d. 25

32. When the patient is positioned for an MLO view, what should be seen on the mammographic image to ensure that the lower posterior breast tissue is seen?

a. The nipple
b. Abdominal tissue
c. Axillary tissue
d. Retromammary space

33. If a patient is concerned about breast discomfort during the procedure, she can be advised to

a. Have the mammogram done right before her period is due.
b. Take an analgesic about an hour before the mammogram is scheduled.
c. Skip the mammogram and have sonography done instead.
d. Wear a sports bra during the exam to minimize compression.

34. Which size plate should be used during MLO positioning for a woman with small breasts?

a. 24 x 30 cm
b. 18 x 24 cm
c. 12 x 18 cm
d. 6 x 12 cm

35. According to the MQSA, what does NOT need to be included on an image label?

a. Facility name
b. Facility location
c. Physician name
d. Patient identification number

36. While developing mammographic film, the technologist notes fog on the image. What is the likely reason for this abnormality?

a. Poor development technique
b. Dust or dirt in the darkroom
c. Light leaking into the room
d. A machine that needs servicing

37. When the skin or nearby fatty tissue appears black, what is the likely source of the problem?

a. Poor technique
b. Underexposure
c. Overexposure
d. Inadequate compression

38. Why is the MLO view preferred over the mediolateral view during routine mammography?

a. The MLO view enables the technician to take a better image of the entire breast, especially the UOQ.
b. There is less discomfort experienced by the patient.
c. It is easier for the technician to take the exposure.
d. There is less radiation exposure for the patient.

39. When taking an MLO image, at what angle should the cassette holder be placed (from the horizontal) for a woman of average height and weight?

a. 20 degrees
b. 30 degrees
c. 45 degrees
d. 60 degrees

40. The technologist should place the woman at what angle to the machine when taking an MLO view?

a. 20 degrees
b. 30 degrees
c. 45 degrees
d. 60 degrees

41. When taking a CC view of the right breast, the technician should stand _____ her when positioning the breast for mammogram.

a. In front of
b. Behind
c. To the right of
d. To the left of

42. When taking a CC view, where should the cassette holder be placed?

a. Above the breast
b. In the inframammary fold
c. Against the axillary tail
d. Against the sternum

43. When taking a mediolateral image, the cassette holder is placed _______ and the compression paddle is placed _________.

a. In the inframammary fold, against the clavicle
b. Against the clavicle, in the inframammary fold
c. Against the sternum, in the axilla
d. In the axilla, against the sternum

44. The technologist is taking a lateromedial image for a diagnostic mammogram. How should she pull the breast to ensure that she gets the proper image?

a. Anteriorly and medially
b. Laterally and medially
c. Superiorly and medially
d. Laterally and anteriorly

45. When taking magnification views, what additional tools does the technologist need to take the proper image?

a. Magnification platform
b. Grid
c. Both of the above
d. Neither of the above

46. When is it appropriate to take a cleavage view?

a. As part of the routine screening mammogram
b. When there is a suspected lesion in the anterior edge of the breast
c. When there is a suspected lesion in the medial or posterior portion of the breasts
d. As a method of spot compression with a suspected lesion in the nipple

47. When taking a caudocranial view, the goal is to visualize tissue in the _______ part of the breast.

a. Lowermost
b. Uppermost
c. Medial
d. Lateral

48. What should be placed on the breast during a tangential view?

a. A compression paddle
b. Grid
c. Lead marker
d. Nothing additional is required

49. A technologist is preparing to perform a mammogram on a woman who has a central venous catheter in place. How should she advise the patient?

a. Tell her the mammogram cannot be done and have her reschedule once the catheter has been removed.
b. Perform the mammogram without any change in procedure.
c. Perform sonography instead of mammography.
d. Consider using a lateromedial oblique view instead of the standard MLO.

50. A patient with a large abdomen is about to have her mammogram. How should the technician advise her?

a. Arch her back and lean into the cassette.
b. Bend over slightly and reduce the angle of the x-ray tube.
c. Angle herself toward the machine at 60 degrees instead of the standard 45 degrees.
d. No changes should be made.

Answer Key and Explanations

1. B: Women should perform monthly breast self-exams beginning at age 20. They should have a physician perform a clinical breast exam every three years (from age 20 to 39 and yearly after that) and a yearly mammogram beginning at age 40. If there is a strong family history of breast or ovarian cancer, clinical breast exams and mammography should be performed more frequently.

2. D: The FDA has not approved breast sonography for use as a routine screening tool. However, it is a useful procedure when a woman is pregnant, has dense breasts or silicone implants, or clarifying lesions are detected during mammography.

3. A: Ductography is indicated when there is abnormal discharge from the nipple. A small amount of contrast material is introduced into a single duct in the nipple, and a mammogram is performed. Choice A describes fine needle aspiration. All of the other choices are correct.

4. B: M*agnetic resonance imaging* (MRI) scans are not appropriate as a routine screening tool and are most useful in showing tumors with increased blood flow or those that are close to the chest wall. They do not show microcalcifications. They should not be performed when a woman is pregnant or has metal in her body (such as a metal pin or rod). They are also contraindicated in patients who are allergic to the contrast material or who are too overweight to fit in the MRI machine.

5. A: Many breast tumors are estrogen dependent, meaning that they grow in the presence of estrogen in the body. Tamoxifen, an estrogen inhibitor, is best used for these estrogen-sensitive tumors. Early menopause and the symptoms associated with menopause (such as osteoporosis) are the side effects of this medication. It should not be used in women who are still planning on pregnancy because of the risk for early menopause.

6. C: A focal spot is where the electrons emerging from the cathode connect with the anode. The focal spot size is related to the location where the x-ray beam is most intense where it strikes the patient. The smaller the angle of the anode, the smaller the size of the focal spot. The large focal spot is usually 0.3 mm; it is used for the majority of mammography. The small focal spot is usually 0.1 mm and is used for more magnified views.

7. B: The film cassette allows the film to be placed as close to the patient as possible and should be allowed to rest for 15 minutes before being exposed to allow all of the air to bleed out of the cassette. If air is not allowed to bleed out of the cassette, the image will be negatively affected.

8. C: Compression force must be maintained between 25 and 45 lbs of force. If routine quality control testing shows the compression force to be out of that range, the machine must be serviced immediately. There must also be a mechanism to release the compression force in the event of power loss.

9. C: Women with thick or dense breasts require a higher dosage of radiation in order for the radiation to be able to penetrate the thick tissue and reach the receptor. Receptors with various levels of sensitivity are available to minimize the increase in dosage, including digital receptors. To maintain appropriate contrast of the image, the peak kilovoltage (kVP) should be decreased, but only to the point that enhances contrast while still allowing penetration of the dense tissue. It is important that technicians be experienced and competent so that they can evaluate the breasts and select the appropriate parameters that will allow minimum exposure time while capturing the most accurate image.

10. B: The AEC, or automatic exposure control, is a sensor found beneath the densest part of the breast and controls exposure length. Electrical energy flows from the anode to the cathode to produce the radiation. The x-ray filter removes excess photons that are not necessary to produce a clear image.

11. C: The source–image distance is the distance from the source of the radiation to the image receptor. The object–image-receptor distance is the distance between the breast and the image receptor. The source–object distance is the distance between the source of the radiation and the breast tissue. The focal-spot–image distance is the distance between the focal spot and the image receptor.

12. B: The grid improves contrast by decreasing radiation scatter. Very thin strips of lead or other metal are placed at a rate of around 60 to 80 strips per centimeter. They absorb extra radiation, thereby reducing scatter. Option A refers to the intensifying screen. Choices C and D are incorrect.

13. A: Dirt and dust particles can contaminate film and produce artifacts on the image. It is extremely important that the darkroom be cleaned each day before developing any film and that any unnecessary items are removed from the darkroom to minimize the risk of contamination.

14. D: A phantom image should be developed and evaluated at least weekly, but also whenever service is performed on the machinery, when the type of film or screen is changed, or to troubleshoot problems.

15. B: The FDA-approved phantom should contain all of the listed characteristics, except that it should be 50% adipose tissue and 50% glandular tissue. The waxy insert should also contain five groups of specks between the diameters of 0.16 and 0.54 mm.

16. D: Unless there is potential for contact with body fluids or moist skin, gloves are sufficient as personal protective equipment (PPE). If there is a risk of coming into contact with body fluids, a gown may be worn over clothes. If going into an isolation room in a hospital, use the PPE as required by your facility for that level of isolation.

17. D: The referring physician should receive a copy of the findings if a malignancy is suspected within 3 to 5 days of the film. Regardless of the result, the patient should also receive a copy of the results within a few days in plain language. If no malignancy is suspected, the referring physician should get the results within 30 days.

18. A: The breast is divided into four quadrants, marked by dividing lines extending through the nipple from the top to the bottom of the breast and across the middle of the breast. Most cancers are found in the upper outer quadrant of the breast, toward the axilla.

19. A: The retromammary space is the space found between the breast tissue and the pectoralis muscle. Fatty or adipose tissue is found in this space. Connective tissue, lymphatic tissue, and fat are also found in the subcutaneous area of the breast. The milk-secreting ducts and lactiferous sinuses are found within the mammary tissue itself.

20. C: The breast is supported by tissue between the second and fourth rib on the vertical plane. It is found between the axilla and the sternum horizontally. Breast tissue extends into the axilla, known as the axillary tail of Spence.

21. D: Approximately 60% of the blood flow to the breast comes from the internal mammary artery, specifically, the anterior perforating branches, which supply the central part of the breast. The upper outer quadrant is supplied by the lateral thoracic artery (approximately 30% of total blood supply). The remainder of the breast is supplied by the thoracoacromial artery, branches of the intercostal arteries, the subcapsular artery, and the thoracodorsal artery.

22. A: There is no muscle tissue within the breast itself. The adipose and connective tissues of the breast sit on top of the pectoralis major muscle on the chest wall. The pectoralis minor muscle is deeper in the chest wall. The mammary muscle is a made-up structure.

23. C: The myoepithelial cells contract to assist in milk ejection from the breast. The luminal cells actually secrete the milk. The luminal cells and myoepithelial cells line the terminal ductal lobular unit (TDLU). The luminal cells are found in the outermost lining of the TDLU, whereas the myoepithelium is the innermost portion of the TDLU lining.

24. A: The Montgomery glands secrete a substance that is thought to protect the delicate areolar and nipple tissue during nursing. The Morgagni tubercles are small outgrowths of the ends of the Montgomery gland ducts. They are found on the edge of the areola. Myoepithelial cells contract and aid in milk ejection from the breast. The alveoli are small structures that conduct milk into the ductal system and eventually out of the nipple.

25. D: A milk-filled cyst is also called a galactocele; it usually results from a blocked milk duct and is a benign lesion. It would appear as an indeterminate mass or a small round or oval lesion with well-defined borders. Galactoceles can occur either during lactation or shortly after.

26. D: Benign calcifications are not cancerous and are usually uniform in mass and density. They tend to have sharp outlines and are well defined. Benign calcifications can be round or oval in shape, although, depending on the type of calcification, they may have a distinct shape, such as pear-shaped (milk of calcium calcification) or ring-shaped (sebaceous gland calcification).

27. B: An eczematous reaction around the areola and nipple indicates Paget's disease. Bleeding or oozing from the nipple is also sometimes seen with Paget's disease. This condition occurs when cancer cells from the original ductal carcinoma migrate through the duct and to the skin of the breast.

28. A: To ensure the best image density (1.5 to 2.0), the exposure time should range between 0.5 and 2.0 seconds. Underexposure reduces contrast and can make it difficult to visualize microcalcifications or other small abnormalities. Overexposure can cause blackening of the skin or fatty tissue and can sometimes be compensated for by illuminating the image with a brighter light source.

29. C: Proper compression of the breast is crucial because it reduces thickness of the breast and ensures even exposure of all of the breast tissue. Proper compression is achieved when the skin is taut and does not dent when a finger is pressed into it. Insufficient compression can cause poor-quality images, and too much compression can actually damage breast tissue and cause pain.

30. B: Compression of the breast allows the x-ray to penetrate the tissue evenly and immobilizes the breast tissue during x-ray exposure. Poor compression can cause poor image contrast and blurring of the image if the breast is not properly immobilized.

31. A: Magnification mammography is usually used to magnify masses and microcalcifications so that they can be more clearly visualized. The image should be magnified between 1.5 and 2.0 times the original image. When performing magnification mammography, a small focal spot (this keeps the borders of the image sharp) and a compression paddle should be used.

32. D: When positioning the patient for a mediolateral-oblique (MLO) view, the entire breast from the pectoralis major muscle through the nipple should be visualized on the image. To make sure that the lower posterior breast tissue is seen, the retromammary space should be visualized on the mammogram.

33. B: Some discomfort is to be expected during a mammogram. More sensitivity is usually reported right before or during a woman's menstrual period, so the test should be scheduled at a different part of the woman's menstrual cycle. She can take an analgesic like ibuprofen or acetaminophen one to two hours before the test. Breast sensitivity is not a reason to skip mammography in favor of sonography. A sports bra should never be worn during the test.

34. B: An 18 x 24 cm plate is usually sufficient for proper compression and image visualization for a woman with small breasts. A larger plate, 24 x 30 cm, is necessary when a woman has larger breasts. Both plates must be available so that the proper instrumentation can be used. The image should be checked before the woman leaves the facility to make sure that it does not need to be retaken.

35. C: According to the Mammography Quality Standards Act (MQSA), the image label should contain the name and location of the facility, patient name and identification number, which breast is on the image, the name of the technician performing the mammogram, the specific x-ray unit performing the mammogram, and the date that the mammogram was taken. The name of the ordering physician does not need to be included on the label.

36. C: Fog on a mammogram usually indicates that light is leaking into the darkroom during development of the film. Dust or dirt in the darkroom causes artifacts on the image. Scratches or fingerprints can indicate problems processing the film or poor development technique. Grid lines appearing on the film usually indicate that the processor or grid is not functioning properly.

37. C: Black skin or nearby fatty tissue usually indicates that the film was overexposed. It can sometimes be corrected by increasing the illumination by which the film is visualized. Underexposure causes the film to have poor contrast and cannot be corrected. The film would need to be repeated.

38. A: The mediolateral-oblique (MLO) view takes an oblique view across the breast and enables more of the upper outer quadrant (UOQ) of the breast to be visualized. More malignancies are found in this quadrant, so it is important that the entire quadrant be visualized during mammography.

39. C: When taking an MLO image, the cassette holder should be placed parallel to the pectoralis major muscle with the edge in the axilla. It should be placed at an angle from the horizontal between 30 and 60 degrees. For a woman of average height and weight, that angle should be between 40 to 50 degrees. For shorter, heavier women, that angle should be lower (between 30 and 40 degrees), and for taller, leaner women, that angle should be higher (between 50 and 60 degrees).

40. C: When taking an MLO view, the woman should be instructed to stand at a 45-degree angle to the machine with her elbow elevated and her hands on the handles. She should be instructed to bend slightly forward at the waist while the technologist positions her breast against the cassette, drawing the medial portion of the breast forward. Once she is in the correct position, compression will be applied.

41. D: When taking a craniocaudal (CC) view, the technician should stand next to the woman on the medial aspect of the breast. If taking an image of the right breast, the medial aspect of the breast points to the left of the patient. The technician should stand on the left-hand side of the woman.

42. B: When taking a craniocaudal view, the cassette holder should be placed in the inframammary fold. The breast should be lifted about 2 cm, and the table (and cassette holder) should be placed underneath it with the nipple in the center.

43 D: When taking a mediolateral view, the image is shot from the middle of the breast outward. The cassette holder should be placed in the axilla, and the compression paddle is placed against the sternum. The breast is pulled anteriorly and medially until the breast tissue is centered against the cassette. This pulls open the inframammary fold.

44. A: When taking a lateromedial view, the image is shot from the side of the breast inward. The cassette holder should be placed against the sternum, and the compression paddle is placed in the axilla. The breast is pulled anteriorly and medially until the breast tissue is centered against the cassette. This pulls open the inframammary fold.

45. A: When taking magnification views, a magnification platform should be placed between the breast tissue and the cassette holder. A grid is not necessary because the platform creates an air gap that prevents scattered radiation from getting to the film.

46. C: A cleavage view is taken when both breasts are placed on the cassette holder after the technologist has slightly elevated both breasts, opening the inframammary fold. This is an appropriate image to take when a suspected lesion is found deep in the medial tissue of the breast.

47. B: A caudocranial view is taken to better see the tissue of the uppermost part of the breasts. The cassette holder is placed on top of the breasts, and the compression paddle is placed below the breasts. This view would also be appropriate for patients suffering from kyphosis, as it would make it easier to see the uppermost tissue that might be missed otherwise.

48. C: A tangential view is best used when a suspected lesion is close to the skin, as the image is taken tangentially to the surface of the skin. A lead marker is placed over the suspected lesion to ensure that the area of concern is noted on the mammogram.

49. D: Technically, the technologist does not need to adjust her technique when taking a mammogram of a patient with a central venous catheter, but she must take care to avoid damaging the catheter or hurting the patient. For that reason, she should consider taking a lateromedial oblique view instead of the standard MLO

50. B: Having a large abdomen may make visualization of the inframammary fold difficult. This can also make compression difficult. The patient should be counseled to bend over slightly, and the technologist should consider reducing the angle of the x-ray tube.

How to Overcome Test Anxiety

Just the thought of taking a test is enough to make most people a little nervous. A test is an important event that can have a long-term impact on your future, so it's important to take it seriously and it's natural to feel anxious about performing well. But just because anxiety is normal, that doesn't mean that it's helpful in test taking, or that you should simply accept it as part of your life. Anxiety can have a variety of effects. These effects can be mild, like making you feel slightly nervous, or severe, like blocking your ability to focus or remember even a simple detail.

If you experience test anxiety—whether severe or mild—it's important to know how to beat it. To discover this, first you need to understand what causes test anxiety.

Causes of Test Anxiety

While we often think of anxiety as an uncontrollable emotional state, it can actually be caused by simple, practical things. One of the most common causes of test anxiety is that a person does not feel adequately prepared for their test. This feeling can be the result of many different issues such as poor study habits or lack of organization, but the most common culprit is time management. Starting to study too late, failing to organize your study time to cover all of the material, or being distracted while you study will mean that you're not well prepared for the test. This may lead to cramming the night before, which will cause you to be physically and mentally exhausted for the test. Poor time management also contributes to feelings of stress, fear, and hopelessness as you realize you are not well prepared but don't know what to do about it.

Other times, test anxiety is not related to your preparation for the test but comes from unresolved fear. This may be a past failure on a test, or poor performance on tests in general. It may come from comparing yourself to others who seem to be performing better or from the stress of living up to expectations. Anxiety may be driven by fears of the future—how failure on this test would affect your educational and career goals. These fears are often completely irrational, but they can still negatively impact your test performance.

Elements of Test Anxiety

As mentioned earlier, test anxiety is considered to be an emotional state, but it has physical and mental components as well. Sometimes you may not even realize that you are suffering from test anxiety until you notice the physical symptoms. These can include trembling hands, rapid heartbeat, sweating, nausea, and tense muscles. Extreme anxiety may lead to fainting or vomiting. Obviously, any of these symptoms can have a negative impact on testing. It is important to recognize them as soon as they begin to occur so that you can address the problem before it damages your performance.

The mental components of test anxiety include trouble focusing and inability to remember learned information. During a test, your mind is on high alert, which can help you recall information and stay focused for an extended period of time. However, anxiety interferes with your mind's natural processes, causing you to blank out, even on the questions you know well. The strain of testing during anxiety makes it difficult to stay focused, especially on a test that may take several hours. Extreme anxiety can take a huge mental toll, making it difficult not only to recall test information but even to understand the test questions or pull your thoughts together.

Effects of Test Anxiety

Test anxiety is like a disease—if left untreated, it will get progressively worse. Anxiety leads to poor performance, and this reinforces the feelings of fear and failure, which in turn lead to poor performances on subsequent tests. It can grow from a mild nervousness to a crippling condition. If allowed to progress, test anxiety can have a big impact on your schooling, and consequently on your future.

Test anxiety can spread to other parts of your life. Anxiety on tests can become anxiety in any stressful situation, and blanking on a test can turn into panicking in a job situation. But fortunately, you don't have to let anxiety rule your testing and determine your grades. There are a number of relatively simple steps you can take to move past anxiety and function normally on a test and in the rest of life.

Physical Steps for Beating Test Anxiety

While test anxiety is a serious problem, the good news is that it can be overcome. It doesn't have to control your ability to think and remember information. While it may take time, you can begin taking steps today to beat anxiety.

Just as your first hint that you may be struggling with anxiety comes from the physical symptoms, the first step to treating it is also physical. Rest is crucial for having a clear, strong mind. If you are tired, it is much easier to give in to anxiety. But if you establish good sleep habits, your body and mind will be ready to perform optimally, without the strain of exhaustion. Additionally, sleeping well helps you to retain information better, so you're more likely to recall the answers when you see the test questions.

Getting good sleep means more than going to bed on time. It's important to allow your brain time to relax. Take study breaks from time to time so it doesn't get overworked, and don't study right before bed. Take time to rest your mind before trying to rest your body, or you may find it difficult to fall asleep.

Along with sleep, other aspects of physical health are important in preparing for a test. Good nutrition is vital for good brain function. Sugary foods and drinks may give a burst of energy but this burst is followed by a crash, both physically and emotionally. Instead, fuel your body with protein and vitamin-rich foods.

Also, drink plenty of water. Dehydration can lead to headaches and exhaustion, especially if your brain is already under stress from the rigors of the test. Particularly if your test is a long one, drink water during the breaks. And if possible, take an energy-boosting snack to eat between sections.

Along with sleep and diet, a third important part of physical health is exercise. Maintaining a steady workout schedule is helpful, but even taking 5-minute study breaks to walk can help get your blood pumping faster and clear your head. Exercise also releases endorphins, which contribute to a positive feeling and can help combat test anxiety.

When you nurture your physical health, you are also contributing to your mental health. If your body is healthy, your mind is much more likely to be healthy as well. So take time to rest, nourish your body with healthy food and water, and get moving as much as possible. Taking these physical steps will make you stronger and more able to take the mental steps necessary to overcome test anxiety.

Mental Steps for Beating Test Anxiety

Working on the mental side of test anxiety can be more challenging, but as with the physical side, there are clear steps you can take to overcome it. As mentioned earlier, test anxiety often stems from lack of preparation, so the obvious solution is to prepare for the test. Effective studying may be the most important weapon you have for beating test anxiety, but you can and should employ several other mental tools to combat fear.

First, boost your confidence by reminding yourself of past success—tests or projects that you aced. If you're putting as much effort into preparing for this test as you did for those, there's no reason you should expect to fail here. Work hard to prepare; then trust your preparation.

Second, surround yourself with encouraging people. It can be helpful to find a study group, but be sure that the people you're around will encourage a positive attitude. If you spend time with others who are anxious or cynical, this will only contribute to your own anxiety. Look for others who are motivated to study hard from a desire to succeed, not from a fear of failure.

Third, reward yourself. A test is physically and mentally tiring, even without anxiety, and it can be helpful to have something to look forward to. Plan an activity following the test, regardless of the outcome, such as going to a movie or getting ice cream.

When you are taking the test, if you find yourself beginning to feel anxious, remind yourself that you know the material. Visualize successfully completing the test. Then take a few deep, relaxing breaths and return to it. Work through the questions carefully but with confidence, knowing that you are capable of succeeding.

Developing a healthy mental approach to test taking will also aid in other areas of life. Test anxiety affects more than just the actual test—it can be damaging to your mental health and even contribute to depression. It's important to beat test anxiety before it becomes a problem for more than testing.

Study Strategy

Being prepared for the test is necessary to combat anxiety, but what does being prepared look like? You may study for hours on end and still not feel prepared. What you need is a strategy for test prep. The next few pages outline our recommended steps to help you plan out and conquer the challenge of preparation.

Step 1: Scope Out the Test

Learn everything you can about the format (multiple choice, essay, etc.) and what will be on the test. Gather any study materials, course outlines, or sample exams that may be available. Not only will this help you to prepare, but knowing what to expect can help to alleviate test anxiety.

Step 2: Map Out the Material

Look through the textbook or study guide and make note of how many chapters or sections it has. Then divide these over the time you have. For example, if a book has 15 chapters and you have five days to study, you need to cover three chapters each day. Even better, if you have the time, leave an extra day at the end for overall review after you have gone through the material in depth.

If time is limited, you may need to prioritize the material. Look through it and make note of which sections you think you already have a good grasp on, and which need review. While you are studying, skim quickly through the familiar sections and take more time on the challenging parts. Write out your plan so you don't get lost as you go. Having a written plan also helps you feel more in control of the study, so anxiety is less likely to arise from feeling overwhelmed at the amount to cover.

Step 3: Gather Your Tools

Decide what study method works best for you. Do you prefer to highlight in the book as you study and then go back over the highlighted portions? Or do you type out notes of the important information? Or is it helpful to make flashcards that you can carry with you? Assemble the pens, index cards, highlighters, post-it notes, and any other materials you may need so you won't be distracted by getting up to find things while you study.

If you're having a hard time retaining the information or organizing your notes, experiment with different methods. For example, try color-coding by subject with colored pens, highlighters, or post-it notes. If you learn better by hearing, try recording yourself reading your notes so you can listen while in the car, working out, or simply sitting at your desk. Ask a friend to quiz you from your flashcards, or try teaching someone the material to solidify it in your mind.

Step 4: Create Your Environment

It's important to avoid distractions while you study. This includes both the obvious distractions like visitors and the subtle distractions like an uncomfortable chair (or a too-comfortable couch that makes you want to fall asleep). Set up the best study environment possible: good lighting and a comfortable work area. If background music helps you focus, you may want to turn it on, but otherwise keep the room quiet. If you are using a computer to take notes, be sure you don't have any other windows open, especially applications like social media, games, or anything else that could distract you. Silence your phone and turn off notifications. Be sure to keep water close by so you stay hydrated while you study (but avoid unhealthy drinks and snacks).

Also, take into account the best time of day to study. Are you freshest first thing in the morning? Try to set aside some time then to work through the material. Is your mind clearer in the afternoon or evening? Schedule your study session then. Another method is to study at the same time of day that you will take the test, so that your brain gets used to working on the material at that time and will be ready to focus at test time.

Step 5: Study!

Once you have done all the study preparation, it's time to settle into the actual studying. Sit down, take a few moments to settle your mind so you can focus, and begin to follow your study plan. Don't give in to distractions or let yourself procrastinate. This is your time to prepare so you'll be ready to fearlessly approach the test. Make the most of the time and stay focused.

Of course, you don't want to burn out. If you study too long you may find that you're not retaining the information very well. Take regular study breaks. For example, taking five minutes out of every hour to walk briskly, breathing deeply and swinging your arms, can help your mind stay fresh.

As you get to the end of each chapter or section, it's a good idea to do a quick review. Remind yourself of what you learned and work on any difficult parts. When you feel that you've mastered the material, move on to the next part. At the end of your study session, briefly skim through your notes again.

But while review is helpful, cramming last minute is NOT. If at all possible, work ahead so that you won't need to fit all your study into the last day. Cramming overloads your brain with more information than it can process and retain, and your tired mind may struggle to recall even previously learned information when it is overwhelmed with last-minute study. Also, the urgent nature of cramming and the stress placed on your brain contribute to anxiety. You'll be more likely to go to the test feeling unprepared and having trouble thinking clearly.

So don't cram, and don't stay up late before the test, even just to review your notes at a leisurely pace. Your brain needs rest more than it needs to go over the information again. In fact, plan to finish your studies by noon or early afternoon the day before the test. Give your brain the rest of the day to relax or focus on other things, and get a good night's sleep. Then you will be fresh for the test and better able to recall what you've studied.

Step 6: Take a Practice Test

Many courses offer sample tests, either online or in the study materials. This is an excellent resource to check whether you have mastered the material, as well as to prepare for the test format and environment.

Check the test format ahead of time: the number of questions, the type (multiple choice, free response, etc.), and the time limit. Then create a plan for working through them. For example, if you have 30 minutes to take a 60-question test, your limit is 30 seconds per question. Spend less time on the questions you know well so that you can take more time on the difficult ones.

If you have time to take several practice tests, take the first one open book, with no time limit. Work through the questions at your own pace and make sure you fully understand them. Gradually work up to taking a test under test conditions: sit at a desk with all study materials put away and set a timer. Pace yourself to make sure you finish the test with time to spare and go back to check your answers if you have time.

After each test, check your answers. On the questions you missed, be sure you understand why you missed them. Did you misread the question (tests can use tricky wording)? Did you forget the information? Or was it something you hadn't learned? Go back and study any shaky areas that the practice tests reveal.

Taking these tests not only helps with your grade, but also aids in combating test anxiety. If you're already used to the test conditions, you're less likely to worry about it, and working through tests until you're scoring well gives you a confidence boost. Go through the practice tests until you feel comfortable, and then you can go into the test knowing that you're ready for it.

Test Tips

On test day, you should be confident, knowing that you've prepared well and are ready to answer the questions. But aside from preparation, there are several test day strategies you can employ to maximize your performance.

First, as stated before, get a good night's sleep the night before the test (and for several nights before that, if possible). Go into the test with a fresh, alert mind rather than staying up late to study.

Try not to change too much about your normal routine on the day of the test. It's important to eat a nutritious breakfast, but if you normally don't eat breakfast at all, consider eating just a protein bar. If you're a coffee drinker, go ahead and have your normal coffee. Just make sure you time it so that the caffeine doesn't wear off right in the middle of your test. Avoid sugary beverages, and drink enough water to stay hydrated but not so much that you need a restroom break 10 minutes into the test. If your test isn't first thing in the morning, consider going for a walk or doing a light workout before the test to get your blood flowing.

Allow yourself enough time to get ready, and leave for the test with plenty of time to spare so you won't have the anxiety of scrambling to arrive in time. Another reason to be early is to select a good seat. It's helpful to sit away from doors and windows, which can be distracting. Find a good seat, get out your supplies, and settle your mind before the test begins.

When the test begins, start by going over the instructions carefully, even if you already know what to expect. Make sure you avoid any careless mistakes by following the directions.

Then begin working through the questions, pacing yourself as you've practiced. If you're not sure on an answer, don't spend too much time on it, and don't let it shake your confidence. Either skip it and come back later, or eliminate as many wrong answers as possible and guess among the remaining ones. Don't dwell on these questions as you continue—put them out of your mind and focus on what lies ahead.

Be sure to read all of the answer choices, even if you're sure the first one is the right answer. Sometimes you'll find a better one if you keep reading. But don't second-guess yourself if you do immediately know the answer. Your gut instinct is usually right. Don't let test anxiety rob you of the information you know.

If you have time at the end of the test (and if the test format allows), go back and review your answers. Be cautious about changing any, since your first instinct tends to be correct, but make sure you didn't misread any of the questions or accidentally mark the wrong answer choice. Look over any you skipped and make an educated guess.

At the end, leave the test feeling confident. You've done your best, so don't waste time worrying about your performance or wishing you could change anything. Instead, celebrate the successful completion of this test. And finally, use this test to learn how to deal with anxiety even better next time.

Review Video: Test Anxiety
Visit mometrix.com/academy and enter code: 100340

Important Qualification

Not all anxiety is created equal. If your test anxiety is causing major issues in your life beyond the classroom or testing center, or if you are experiencing troubling physical symptoms related to your anxiety, it may be a sign of a serious physiological or psychological condition. If this sounds like your situation, we strongly encourage you to seek professional help.

Online Resources

Due to our efforts to try to keep this book to a manageable length, we've created a link that will give you access to all of your online resources:

mometrix.com/resources719/mammography

It's Your Moment, Let's Celebrate It!

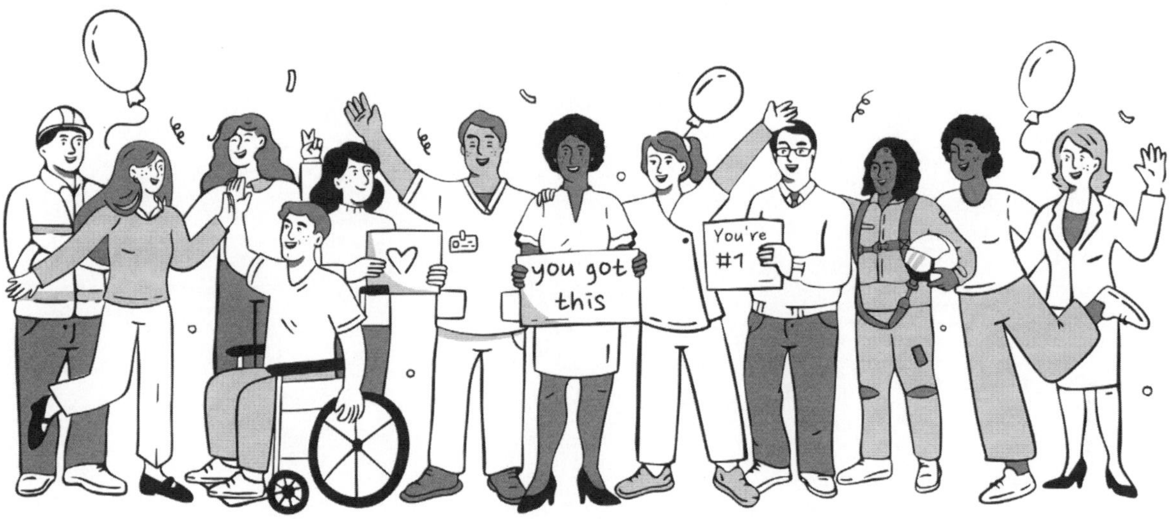

Share your story @mometrixtestpreparation